THE SILENT SYNDROME:

Women and Doctors Reveal How Routine Medical Procedures Cause Infertility, Miscarriages and Asherman's Syndrome

Compiled and edited by Corinna Maria Dartenne
and Poly Spyrou

With an Introduction by Poly Spyrou,
Founder of the International Asherman´s Association

Many thanks to all the women who provided their stories for this book; to all those who, read, wrote, offered comments and assisted in the editing, proofreading and design of this book.

A special thanks to Anoka Faruqee for volunteering to head this project and put the book together and even paid out of pocket for an assistant to help her.

TABLE OF **CONTENTS**

PREFACE: Anoka Faruqee 7

FOREWORD: Sophie Blake: The Silent Syndrome............11

INTRODUCTION: Poly Spyrou: The Accidental Activist 15

I: TRYING TO CONCEIVE 23

    1. Lorie...24

    2. Anoka: Learning from Loss 29

    3. Doreen 39

    4. Karen 43

    5. Rhonda 49

**II: POST-ASHERMAN'S PREGNANCY
AND CHILDBIRTH**...55

    6. Christy 57

    7. Lucila 59

    8. Corinna: The Power of Online Support Groups 69

    9. Jennifer F. 77

    10. Jennifer G. 83

    11. Sue 93

    12. Jennifer H. A Miracle of Tiniest Proportions 97

    13. Paige. 103

    14. Paula 107

    15. Mandy 113

    16. Susan 119

    17. Leanne 125

    18. Lauren 129

    19. Laura 137

20. Andrea...147

21. Karina 151

22. Kathy 155

III: ADOPTION...**171**

23. Theresa 173

24. Darlene 179

IV: MOVING ON...**187**

25. Louise 189

26. Amanda 197

27. Sonia 205

28. Stacey 215

29. Kay...225

30. Heather 241

31. Coba 249

32. JF 265

VI: DOCTOR'S PERSPECTIVE **275**

33. Paul Indman 277

34. Keith Isaacson 289

35. Charles March 295

36. Dave Olive 311

37. Thierry Vancaillie 319

PREFACE

Anoka Faruqee

Routine medical procedures such as dilation and curettage (D&C) and other typical uterine surgeries carry a terrifying risk: infertility. These surgeries for fibroids, miscarriage, elective abortion, or retained placenta after a complicated delivery can scar or damage the lining of the uterus, creating web-like scar tissue or adhesions that cause the uterine lining to stick to itself or close completely, effectively making it impossible for a woman to get pregnant or carry a pregnancy to term without treatment. This devastating condition is called Asherman's Syndrome. The most common and untrue assertion about Asherman's is that it is rare. Current data shows quite the opposite, with a frequency of Asherman's as high as 30% after postpartum D&Cs. Alarmingly, most doctors do not inform patients of, or even acknowledge, these real risks of infertility, recurrent miscarriage, and complicated pregnancies. Rather, doctors often present these sometimes unnecessary procedures, used for several purposes, as harmless panaceas. No one hears of Asherman's Syndrome until she actually suffers from the condition. *The Silent Syndrome* is a collection of stories from women and doctors, many of whom have never met in person but who formed a vibrant, international, online community to fill a devastating void: the staggering lack of information about the real risks of uterine surgeries. This is a crucial manuscript for all couples who want children and every doctor who treats them.

The women in this volume suffered from infertility; in seeking solutions, they gained knowledge and informed their own physicians. These are stories of loss, disbelief, and grief, but with turning points of renewed resilience in the face of injustice and hardship. Each woman's story represents various stages of the condition in breathtakingly real, first-person voice. No detail is spared—good, bad, or ugly. Though many of these chapters resolve in successful live births, others take the reader through the experiences of adoption or the brave journey of coming to terms with not having children after many unsuccessful attempts at medical recovery.

The unique, hybrid format presents women's vivid personal voices alongside objective medical scholarship. Perspectives from the world's leading fertility doctors provide much-needed expertise on prevention, diagnosis, and treatment. Written for a lay audience, the doctors' contributions substantiate the very real threat of Asherman's Syndrome, which is largely underdiagnosed. Our hope is that these approachable essays will ultimately lead to patient awareness, further research, and the development of best practices in the medical community. For example, readers will be surprised to learn that most D&Cs are performed blindly: the doctor places a curette (a scoop shaped surgical instrument) inside the uterus to remove tissue, but he/she cannot see inside to accurately control its placement or action. Doctors in this volume propose an alternative— visualized surgery aided by ultrasound or hysteroscope—as a simple move in the right direction. Furthermore, several doctors in this volume suggest that simple and safe prophylactic measures—such as a temporary uterine stent to prevent scarring and high-dose estrogen therapy to promote endometrial growth and healing—could greatly reduce the risk of uterine adhesions and preserve the fertility of thousands of women.

This book would not exist without the courageous efforts of Poly Spyrou, who founded Ashermans.org more than a decade ago and continues to provide the tireless vision and leadership that brings this online Asherman's community together. Ashermans.org is now a non-profit organization working to educate women across the globe about Asherman's

Syndrome. Poly Spyrou rightly decided that for too many years women with intrauterine scarring had suffered in ignorance and silence. A remarkable collective memoir, this book is a testament to her unbreakable spirit.

FOREWORD

Sophie Blake

THE SILENT SYNDROME

If the Silent Syndrome had been written a few years ago it could have personally spared me a lot of personal heartache and pain. It could have prevented a long 21 month battle to get diagnosed with Asherman´s Syndrome after the birth of my daughter. Like most people, I had never heard of it. No one warned me that the so called simple procedure used to manually remove my retained placenta (a blind D&C) after my daughter´s birth could cause me to become infertile. I spent months sitting at the desks of different doctors asking why my periods hadn't returned, why I was in so much pain every month and why I couldn't get pregnant again, only to be constantly brushed aside. Eventually I did my own research and asked if it was possible that I had internal scar tissue. I was told, like so many other women, that it was impossible and incredibly rare. This is a common phrase used by doctors and specialists when discussing AS as shockingly so many are unaware of it or the risk that "simple" uterine surgery can cause.

Asherman´s Syndrome is mainly caused through routine D&C's and surgery for fibroids, miscarriage, elective abortions or the removal of a retained placenta. It can make it impossible for a woman to get pregnant or to stay pregnant without treatment. Devastatingly it goes largely undiagnosed so many women suffer the heartbreak of infertility or recurrent miscarriage's without ever knowing why.

Women are not warned of the dangers or risks that are involved in these surgeries. Asherman´s Syndrome can rob women of their fertility and yet it can easily be prevented if more people are made aware of it and how to prevent it. Many women, like myself, have to turn to the Internet to self-diagnose and yet startlingly there is a serious lack of information out there. This is why an incredible woman called Poly Spyrou, herself a sufferer of AS, founded Ashermans.org over 10 years ago. It is now a thriving on-line community with thousands of members from around the world supporting each other and sharing information to help them get through their Asherman's journey. The support from these women was and is still invaluable to me. They helped see me through my darkest moments and I will be eternally grateful to them all.

It was through this community that I managed to get myself diagnosed and finally see a top specialist in the UK. My beautiful daughter was born in May 2007. Her birth was followed by two manual removals for a retained placenta. My periods failed to ever return (aside from the occasional dark blemish) and yet every month I was in constant pain with a huge swollen stomach. For a few days of each month I would be in a great amount of discomfort, unable to even walk or sit properly without being in great pain. Yet this never set any alarm bells off to the numerous specialists I saw, even when I told them the history of the delivery. As each month after her birth passed, the pain just got worse and worse. My partner Scott and I started trying for another baby when our daughter was 1 but I never fell pregnant. Hormone tests showed I was ovulating so the doctors I saw just said my periods would return at some point and to keep on trying. Finally in February 2009 my local hospital finally performed a laparoscopy and hysteroscopy to see what was going on. The results were devastating. My womb was totally scarred together and the adhesions had grown solidly across my cervix. I had been ovulating and having periods but they were trapped inside each month causing all the pain. They told me that nothing could be done and that the only way to ever have another child was to use a surrogate. I found the Asherman's site that very same day and found my AS specialist, Mr. Lower, through it. He is one of only a handful in the UK. Unfortunately by the time he saw me my AS had become one of the worst cases he had seen. The long wait to get diagnosed meant that a huge amount of damage had been caused to my uterus. I had numerous hysteroscopies and treatments with him but my scar tissue grew back at an alarmingly aggressive rate. We tried a round of IVF in Sept 2009 but that too failed. We heart brokenly resigned ourselves to the fact that we would never have another child naturally and grieved for what could have been. What got us through it was knowing how fortunate we were to already have our daughter.

Anyone facing infertility issues knows how exhausting and emotionally draining it is trying to conceive and then facing up to the fact that the journey is over. We decided to give ourselves some time before deciding whether to continue our desire to complete our family through surrogacy or adoption. Incredibly during this time, I became pregnant. At first we were too scared and shocked to be excited but as the weeks rolled by and the scans came through indicating no serious problems, we started to let our guards down and plan for the future with our miracle baby. Tragically though it wasn't meant to be. At 15 weeks I had an uncontrollable hemorrhage. The doctors desperately tried to save mine and the baby´s life but eventually we were given the horrific news that they would have to remove the baby to save my life. I had placenta previa caused by the placenta growing too low. This in turn was caused by the damage the AS had done to my uterus. It was the most traumatic and devastating experience of my life and one that I could never repeat. My battle with AS still isn't over as I faced two more D&C's after losing the baby and it has returned. However, my battle to conceive another baby naturally is over.

The Silent Syndrome contains a collection of stories from many brave inspiring women who have suffered from the heartbreak of discovering they have AS. Each face the AS fight full of resolve and strength determined to win the AS fight and have a child. Many go on to have successful treatment and thankfully there are many much loved post AS babies out there. This is thanks to the wonderful specialists and determination of these women. Others, like myself, aren't so fortunate but some go on to complete their families through surrogacy or adoption. There are also the perspectives from the world leading fertility doctors who provide much needed expertise on prevention, diagnosis and treatment.

Raising awareness of this Syndrome is vitally important, not just to patients but to the whole medical community. I am still so amazed and disappointed that I have to explain what my "condition" is to those in the medical field, many of whom who work in fertility!

The information and courageous stories in here could have prevented my own AS battle. I truly hope that The Silent Syndrome goes onto book cases everywhere so that women no longer have to suffer such a preventable heartbreaking Syndrome. The fertility of thousands of women could be spared.

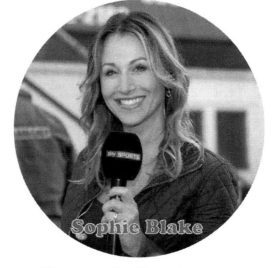

Photo credit: Chris Simpson

INTRODUCTION

Poly Spyrou, Founder of the Online Asherman's Community

THE ACCIDENTAL ACTIVIST

My story starts with personal tragedy but ends with collective empowerment. Out of my trauma came the basic human need to connect with other women to share my grief and keep my sanity. And out of that community ultimately came information and understanding about a Syndrome that a doctor in my country of Cyprus didn't even know how to spell.

After thirteen years of fertility issues, my husband and I tried a new and improved in vitro fertilization (ICSI) and, incredibly, it worked. At thirty-six, after five IVFs, I was finally pregnant, with twins. We planned to name one of the boys Panayiotis, after the Virgin Mary's name "Panayia," and the other Theodoros, meaning "God's gift." But, at twenty-three weeks, I went into early labor. Panayiotis was born first, at 6:05 a.m. I heard him cry and they quickly brought him over to me, then rushed him upstairs to the neonatal department. Theodoros was born at 6:20 a.m. I understood from the way the doctors huddled around him and murmured quietly that he was not going to survive. I took a breath and spoke. I told them that I knew he was dead but that I still wanted to see him. They said that first I had to have the placenta removed via dilation and curettage (D&C), a surgical procedure that uses a curette to scrape out the contents of the uterus.

I found out later that the umbilical cord had been tied around Theodoros' neck. He lived for just a few minutes and then left this world. After the surgery, they brought my sweet, lost Theodoros to me in a bundle of green surgical cloth. A nurse held him in front of me: he was a beautiful baby and just looked like he was sleeping. I was too drowsy from anesthesia to think straight, and to this day I regret not holding him.

While my family was at Theodoros' funeral, I was alone in a hospital room with happy, smiling pregnant women and little babies. I grew deeply depressed. I wanted so desperately to go see Panayiotis. As I entered the neonatal intensive care unit (NICU), the first thing that caught my attention was the sound coming out of the incubators. Bells rang constantly, each one attached to monitors on babies inside the incubators. I was shocked to see Panayiotis surrounded by wires from his tiny head to his tinier toes. He had a tube in his nose to send oxygen to his lungs. He was so small, yet seemed quite long. All his toes and fingers were perfectly formed, but his eyes were bandaged to prevent him from looking into the light above him. I wanted so much to touch him, but he was too fragile, and I didn't want to do anything that might lessen his chances of survival. I visited Panayiotis twice a day every day that I was in the hospital.

After the delivery, I noticed there were liver-like pieces falling out of me. I informed a nurse, but she dismissed it as normal. After ten days, just before being released from the hospital, I felt a great pain in my stomach while sitting on the toilet. As I stood up, I grew dizzy and faint. I held onto the wall and inched out of the stall to call for help, but my voice failed me. Somehow I managed to make it back into my room and onto my bed, just as I was blacking out. When the nurse finally arrived she stuck two pillows under my feet and said I would be fine. I soon felt much better and my husband Kyriaco took me home.

But the next day I grew feverish. The days passed with great pain. I finally convinced the doctors to take my case seriously, and I was soon back in the hospital with a severe infection. I secretly read my hospital notes when the file was left at the end of my bed, which was how I found out that they had left placenta inside me. It was like some big secret. My body was growing ill with sepsis while trying to expel it. As the placenta rotted inside me, a foul smell developed and the pieces continued to fall out of my body. The placenta had to be removed as soon as possible, via another D&C. With my newborn baby in the NICU struggling to survive, the last thing on my mind was how these two curettages might affect my future fertility. Every hour Panayiotis was out of my sight, I missed him terribly. Nurses brought an antibiotic drip, but I wanted to see my baby first.

I was not prepared for how his condition had worsened in less than a day. He had begun to turn black. An infection caused poor circulation and was slowly killing him. But the bandages were off his eyes, and I believe he could feel my presence because he turned his gaze toward me. "My beautiful baby, what is happening to you? I'm so sorry." I felt so guilty; I had failed miserably to keep him inside me and then failed again to keep him away from outside infections. I stroked his little body, sent him a kiss with my fingers, then left.

Around 9 o'clock that night, recovering after the curettage, I had a sudden urge to go see Panayiotis once more. I needed to be escorted by a nurse, but they were all too busy. At that exact time, Kyriaco received a call from the hospital saying that Panayiotis was going to die and asking if he would like to see him. He said no, and he also told them not to tell me. I guess he was in a state of shock. My maternal instincts were so powerful that I could feel my son calling me and I didn't listen. Panayiotis died alone, just three weeks old. In the morning, from the look on Kyriaco's face, I knew that our second baby had died. In all of our years together, I had never seen Kyriaco cry until then. I wasn't able to summon tears. I was too numb with shock. It was all over.

Memories of visiting Panayiotis came to my mind. Every day before I visited him, I would go to a small hospital chapel beside the NICU and I would drop to my knees and pray for him. Because I wanted to be humble, I would pray for all the other babies and children in the hospital first, and only at the end pray for Panayiotis. Kyriaco prayed too in his own way, promising that if Panayiotis's life was spared he would spend time in a monastery and would walk to the monastery on his hands and knees to show his humbleness. He lost his faith the day Panayiotis died.

Panayiotis was baptized the same day he was born. So Panayiotis, unlike Theodoros, was privileged with a church reception at his funeral.
Our plan had been to restart IVF immediately, but we couldn't begin until my periods returned. When they didn't return after the twins' birth, I had a diagnostic hysteroscopy, in which my doctor inserted a small camera into my uterus. He found that the D&C procedures had caused severe scarring that had made the sides of my uterus stick together like a flat pancake. At the time I didn't understand the severity of my case. The doctors didn't want to answer my questions—they simply said that I needed more surgery. I trusted them, especially when one of the doctors insisted that my case was particularly difficult and that his colleague was the sole doctor in Cyprus capable of performing this kind of surgery. So into the surgery room I went again for my third surgery in four months.

When I came out of the surgery, I was told straight out that my uterus was irreparable and that I would need a surrogate if Kyriaco and I wanted a biological child of our own. I don't think I could have heard a crueler diagnosis. After so many years of fertility issues and losing my babies, this diagnosis was too much to bear. The doctor just sat there and shook his head negatively when I asked if I could get help in another country. He played with his pen, waiting for me to pay for the surgery so he could see his next patient. As I was nearly out the door, I turned and asked if what I had been diagnosed with had a name. He gave me a piece of paper with the words "Usheman's Syndrome" on it, admitting that he didn't know if that was the correct spelling. At least I had something to begin my search with.

I spent hours online researching that night. I discovered that the correct spelling was *Asherman's*, but other than that, it was difficult to find any information. I couldn't believe my bad luck. Could Asherman's really be so rare that no one ever talked or wrote about it? I refused to believe that I was the only person in the world suffering from this Syndrome. I spent thirteen nights and days researching on the Internet, determined to find something. The more I searched the angrier I became. Nothing of any value came up.

Meanwhile, I was involved in an online support group for women who had lost multiple births, which gave me both comfort and encouragement. I think I would have gone mad if these virtual friendships hadn't been there for me. Then, suddenly, it clicked: if I couldn't find information on the Internet about Asherman's, I would create a support group for Asherman's just like the one I was in, and women would eventually find their way to it. It was December of 1999. My original plan had been to celebrate the best Christmas ever while pregnant, looking forward to the year 2000 and life with the twins after that. But instead of a Christmas tree that year, I just bought a pair of gold angel faces in memory of my boys. I was mourning the loss of my babies, my dreams, and now my fertility. What did I have to celebrate?

So on December 26, 1999, while everyone else was in the Christmas spirit, I began researching how to properly create a Yahoo group. After about a month, I connected to another woman online in a health forum who was also suffering from Asherman's. I invited her to my new group, and we began e-mailing. I began leaving messages on all the health forums, inviting women who had any connection with Asherman's to join. By the end of February 2000, we had ten members. It was exciting to find others in situations like my own, but our knowledge was still so limited, and none of the women had been treated successfully or gone on to have a baby.

Around the same time, I started exploring adoption. Of course, I still hoped that I would find a doctor who could help me and a treatment that would work, but I needed to have a plan B. I also began to take legal action against the hospital that treated me so badly. I gathered up all the information I had and went to a well-known lawyer who, a year later, managed to settle my case out of court. I also asked the head of the obstetrics department to send me abroad for additional treatment. Unfortunately, the doctor I saw in the United Kingdom punctured my uterus during surgery, which led to more invasive surgery—a laparoscopy as well as a hysteroscopy to repair the damage. After the surgery, he said he had some bad news for me. For a moment I thought he was going to say that he had removed my uterus, so it was a relief to find out that I still had one. We had to return to the United Kingdom for a follow-up after a month, which turned into another surgery. My scarring had returned.

In July 2002, we adopted our daughter, Mariam, from the republic of Georgia. I fell in love with her instantly. She was four months and three weeks old when I first met her, but she was so tiny. I never believed that I could love another child so much again after giving birth to my own biological children. Mariam changed all that.

In the meantime, my online group was slowly growing, and the support I received from the women in the group helped me survive. They cheered me on when I went for surgery in the United Kingdom, prayed for my healing after it was unsuccessful, and gave me hope when I had lost my own. In our group I met Corinna, from Germany, who offered her home to me while I had surgery with a doctor in her country who had successfully treated her. I traveled alone to a country I had never before been to, stayed with a woman whom I knew only from the Internet, and had surgery with a doctor whom I had never met. Some people would have thought me mad, but the trust we built within our group was so strong. Unfortunately, the results were the same as before—more scarring and another uterine puncture.

As the group grew, so did our shared understanding of Asherman's. We started archiving our hard-fought for knowledge, and compiling questions and answers for new members. As names of doctors were mentioned, we collected their information and created an "A-list" of doctors whose surgeries allowed many women from our group to move on to successful births. We were also making a difference in the medical community. I was asked to coauthor a doctor's conference abstract on Asherman's Syndrome using data we had compiled on each woman in the group. And during a medical conference in the United States, we helped bring together eight of the A-listers to discuss possible joint research on Asherman's. One of my proudest achievements occurred in 2007, when we arranged for an A-lister in the United States to come to Cyprus to perform surgery on twenty-seven women, mostly from Cyprus, but also from Portugal, Greece, Turkey, and the United Kingdom.

Some amazing stories have arisen out of this group: stories of women who were given no hope by their doctors but ended up with babies, and stories of women who moved on to adoption or surrogacy only to find themselves pregnant. Twenty-four hours a day, all around the world, we were there for each other. No e-mail was left unanswered. We had become a family.

But 2007 was bittersweet for me. That year marked my eighth and last surgery, my final attempt to restore my uterus. Unfortunately, too many mistakes had taken place, and my chance of carrying a child again was gone. Only a day after that final surgery, I found myself standing in front of a group of doctors and patients, giving a speech at a seminar to create awareness of Asherman's among doctors in Cyprus. I knew that I had to tell my story, but I had never stood up and spoken in front of an audience. I was so nervous, but I felt empowered knowing that more than 1,000 members in the group were behind me.

I continue to moderate the Asherman's group, which can have upward of seventy-five posts a day. I skim each post, and if any goes unanswered, I forward it to other women who may be able to respond. We have several new members every week, and each time a new member joins, we ask her to fill out an Excel spreadsheet detailing her Asherman's history. Each time I read of a change in a member's status, such as a surgery or pregnancy, I contact her to update her files. We have nearly 1,800 patient files in our database. As women have become more active on the site, several have gone on to start their own sites and blogs. Our underdiagnosed and submerged Syndrome is finally rising to the surface. People are becoming aware that it exists, and women finally have a place to go to obtain information, support, and direction. In addition to the Yahoo support group, we have created a general informational website, www.ashermans.org Volunteer members built the site, maintain the files, and manage the group. Both of these forums have changed the lives of many women around the world. We also have our own support group on Facebook. Finally, now we are seeing the diagnosis and successful treatment of many women. If we continue to tell our stories, eventually prevention will prevail, so other women won't have to suffer as I did.

I. TRYING TO CONCEIVE

1. LORIE

My daughter Emalyn Jewel was born on June 16th, 2008. It took my doctor forty-five minutes to manually extract my placenta. I called my doctor´s office twice in regards to the bleeding afterwards and the woman in the office said it was normal. When I had my six-week postpartum check up in late July, I was still bleeding heavily. After an ultrasound, the OB/GYN office scheduled me for a D&C for retained placenta almost two months after my delivery. In the recovery room after the surgery, I was in severe pain. I asked the nurses repeatedly if it was normal to be in this much pain and all of them said it was. They gave me more pain medicine and sent me home.

At home, I was still in severe pain. I called everyone I knew that had had a D&C and asked them if it was normal to have so much pain. Everyone said no. In the bathroom, the whole toilet filled with blood. My husband got a hold of the doctor who said that both the pain and blood were completely normal: she called in three prescriptions: for infection, uterine contractions and pain. I was in so much pain that I was curled up in a ball crying that something was wrong. I remember it like it was yesterday. It was stabbing pain. I couldn't breathe or talk, it was so bad. It felt like something was tearing inside over and over again and every second it got worse. My husband called the doctor´s office again and left a message. Before the doctor could call me back however I had called 911 and was already in our local emergency room.

At the hospital, they did a CT scan and found a perforated uterus. My doctor wanted me transported back to where the D&C was performed to be under her care. I sat in pain all night without any answers: the doctor never came to evaluate my situation. They had sent my husband home and told him to come back in the morning. There were no doctors coming until the next day, so I begged the nurses for more pain medicine but they wouldn't call the doctor for more medication orders.

Finally the next morning the doctor came to see me. She told me that a perforated uterus would usually heal itself. She said that I could wait it out or have her do an exploratory laparoscopy. I told her that something else had to be wrong because of all pain I was having. I was so angry that no one was listening to me.

During the laparoscopy she had found that I had a perforated uterus and that things still didn't look right in there so she called in the general surgeon to take a look. The general surgeon agreed, and opened me up. He found that I did in fact have a perforated bowel which resulted in an emergency bowel resection, appendectomy, and uterus repair. I had twenty-one staples from my bellybutton down, four inches of my small bowel removed, two inch laceration of my uterus which required stitches, and I was in the hospital for eight days without being able to see my two month old daughter. I was so depressed that they ended up having to call in a counselor to see me. I cried for all eight days I was there. That was only the start of all of my problems.

Both doctors had told me that everything went well and by no means would my health be compromised in any way. But to date, I have been diagnosed with chronic abdominal pain Syndrome for all of the adhesions that have formed in my bowels. I get episodes at least three times a month where I get this raw pain in my stomach where it hurts to even walk or bend over. It lasts constantly for three or four days straight. Nothing I do makes it go away. I will be in pain for the rest of my life and am dealing with a pain management plan set up by my gastrointestinal doctor. If that doesn't work, he recommends lyses of the adhesions, which will most likely result in more adhesions of my bowels. Lyses of adhesions require more surgery. They would have to either laparoscopically go in, or open me up due to excessive scar tissue, and remove the adhesions with a laser. The success rate for that is minimal because every time there is surgery or trauma to your abdominal cavity you are at risk for new adhesions to form.

I have been to three obstetricians and have been diagnosed with Asherman's Syndrome by all three. I also may have developed endometriosis because of the Asherman´s Syndrome. Both have affected my fertility. I am still in the process finding out how to repair my fertility, and looking for a doctor I feel comfortable to treat me. Not many doctors around here have knowledge of Asherman´s and how to treat it. I feel like I am going in circles. One of the doctors told me the scar tissue is low and to go ahead and try to conceive. If I can't conceive on my own he would do an intrauterine insemination. So we tried to conceive for six months and have not been successful. It looks like I will have to have surgery to remove the scar tissue in my uterus. She seems to think that it will also help with the adhesion pain I get when I get my period or ovulate.

Surgery is a really hard thing for me to do. I have been seeing a therapist who diagnosed me with post traumatic stress disorder. I have dreams at least three times a month where I am laying on the operating table watching the doctors play with my intestines while I'm trying to talk to them; they can't hear anything I am saying. I wake up soaking wet with sweat and cannot fall asleep afterwards. Going to doctors, thinking about surgeries, or even what happened to me sets off severe panic attacks. When I get my panic attacks, I fear of passing out. I have passed out a few times from them. It starts with a racing heart. Then I feel like I can't breathe or catch my breath. It's so scary. From there my symptoms magnify. I get really hot and dizzy. I usually have to go outside or splash my face to help me calm down. It usually lasts for ten minutes. Then for hours afterwards I feel detached from my body, like living in a bubble. I could get five or ten panic attacks in a day, for days on end. Sometimes it gets so bad I'm afraid to leave my house. I need to heal mentally before going ahead with this surgery. I know it is what I have to do. No one said that this journey on earth would be easy. Hopefully I will be able to beat this Asherman's and hold another sweet angel in my arms.

2. ANOKA

LEARNING FROM LOSS

At age thirty-six, I became pregnant for the first time easily. An ultrasound at six weeks revealed that I had a "blighted ovum," a situation where a fertilized egg implants itself into the uterine wall but the embryo does not develop, leaving an empty sac. I was completely heartbroken; my doctor told me it was just "bad luck." My options, according to my obstetrician, were to have a D&C (dilation and curettage), a surgical procedure that uses suction to empty the uterus, or allow my body to miscarry naturally. She presented the D&C as a routine procedure with limited risks: a 1 percent risk of piercing my uterus versus a very small risk of infection if I miscarried naturally. My husband and I decided to go for the D&C at nine and a half weeks of the pregnancy. Stunned by the unexpected loss, I wanted to move on and start trying to get pregnant again as soon as possible. The D&C was quick and physically painless.

Six weeks after the procedure, my period returned with two, instead of my usual four, days of menstrual flow. When my period was over, I thought, "Is that it?" Several months later, my periods were still light, and I wasn't pregnant. A friend who had pursued fertility treatments gave me the number of her acupuncturist. On the phone, this acupuncturist mentioned that some of her clients had trouble building their uterine linings after a D&C. I was taken aback at the first mention that a D&C could affect my fertility in any way.

I went back to see the same doctor who performed the D&C to describe my short period. Her face grew pale and she mentioned for the first time that some women have scarring of the uterus after several D&C's; however, she didn't put me in this category because I was still getting periods and had had only one D&C. When my blood tests revealed normal hormonal levels, she sent me home to keep trying for two more months and then come back. I never did return to see her, though months later I sent her an incisive letter detailing her negligence.

I went to a second obstetrician to measure my uterine lining via ultrasound, and it was six millimeters (considered on the thin side), not likely to support implantation of an embryo and very likely to result in miscarriage. I said to my sister, "I hope I'm not pregnant." But later that same month I saw floaters and felt faint during a yoga class. I knew from my reading on acupuncture that floaters can signal pregnancy. Occasionally the liver cannot adequately supply blood to the uterus and the eyes at the same time, which reduces blood flow to the optical nerve, creating floaters. I tested the next morning; the egg had begun to implant enough to create the pregnancy hormone and show up on a home pregnancy test at thirteen days past ovulation. But the test result would soon reverse. I tested again each day for the next five days, watching as the test line faded along with my spirit. Eventually the line disappeared and I got a crampier period than usual.

I googled "chemical pregnancy," the unfriendly term for this kind of very early pregnancy loss. It led me to *failed implantation*, which led me to *uterine abnormalities*, which led me to *adhesions*, which led me to the Wikipedia page of *Asherman's Syndrome* and Ashermans.org. I remember that search sequence vividly and how my heart sank in fear and debilitating regret when I read the Wikipedia page. I did not want to believe that I might have uterine scarring that would cause infertility. I wished desperately that I had taken the natural route and avoided the D&C. Could it be possible that this choice, based mostly on convenience and expediency, might prevent me from ever having children? I read in disbelief that the risks of scarring after D&C were much higher than I could have imagined and that the only treatment was more surgery. It was not a doctor, but my body and the Internet that led me to this information. Then a hysterosalpingogram (HSG) X-ray test, where a contrast dye is injected into the uterus and fallopian tubes, revealed a uterine cavity with "two small linear filling defects," which signaled adhesions in the uterus, confirming what my body was already telling me. Even if I was not the classic extreme case, I had Asherman's Syndrome.

Western medicine deals in black and white while Chinese medicine accounts for all the subtle shades of gray in between. Fertility challenges come in many shades of gray. Traditional Chinese medicine became an emotional pillar in my life. It opened my eyes to a new way of approaching my body: to pay attention to and trust it. My acupuncturist asked me about the color, quantity, and quality of my menstrual blood, signs that indicate overall uterine health. Optimally, menstruation should be mostly bright-red periods (the color of a cut), at least four days of real flow, and have very few clots. I also paid attention to skin, hair, and digestion. Because I had always had dry skin, dry hair, was prone to allergies, and often felt colder than other people, the acupuncturist determined that I probably had "blood deficiency," or a lower blood volume. This Chinese medicine diagnosis did not mean that I was clinically ill, just that on a very subtle level I had this challenge.

After several months of acupuncture, exercise, taking herbs, and eating a modified diet, my period increased from two to three days. I altered my already healthy diet to eliminate refined sugars, refined grains, and some dairy products. I ate a mostly organic "blood-building" diet of foods rich in iron, folic acid, vitamin C, and B12. Blood deficiency often leads to "blood stasis" or poor circulation. Gentle exercise and abdominal massage is key for getting blood to the uterus, as are a number of supplements that increase blood flow, such as low-dose aspirin and CoQuinone. I attended a five day retreat run by a well-known fertility acupuncturist and author with a group of women struggling with fertility. We sought calm and spiritual sustenance to steward our futures and heal our bodies. We learned, paradoxically, that to be receptive to new life, we ultimately had to let go of our monomaniacal pregnancy goals. Though we had to be "yang" (motivated, powerful, active), we also needed to nurture "yin" (introspective, nurturing, calm). Yin and yang deficiencies can lead to physical symptoms of imbalance. The acupuncturist quoted Taoist philosophy: "Instead of being the person who climbs the mountain, be the valley so the universe comes to you."

After the retreat, I went to see a leading Asherman's specialist whom I had been referred to by one of the acupuncturists I met. After looking at my HSG X-ray images, he confirmed that I had a mild case of Asherman's and believed that the chemical pregnancy was a result of the scarring. I would need to use birth control for the time being due to the likelihood of another miscarriage. He claimed he could remove the scar tissue via hysteroscopic surgery, in which a small camera would be inserted into my uterus. He was confident, but I was hesitant. My mistrust of the Western medical community and fear of all uterine procedures, even diagnostic ones, were very real. I had taken refuge in alternative medicine in part as an act of political resistance: a response to the injustice of the D&C. I had been robbed of my fertility needlessly and that was a violation of my basic human rights.

I joined the online Asherman's Yahoo group, and within seconds of posting my introduction to the group, I got a response from a woman in my home city of Los Angeles who had experienced four miscarriages, been diagnosed with Asherman's, and had sought the same type of treatment from the very same doctor. Here immediately was a kindred spirit of circumstance—someone I could meet for tea and talk to. Many other women in the group were already chatting about this same specialist and his success rate with corrective surgery, and the superiority of his micro-scissor surgery over laser surgery. They were simultaneously using specialized medical acronyms (RPOC, HSG, SHG) and chatspeak (OMG, LOL!) with equal ease. There were so many voices and so much valuable information. Like a storybook character stepping into a secret doorway, a new world of empathy and knowledge opened up to me. With it came what seemed like a whole new type of communication, with women who were at once strangers and instant friends. I was hooked.

I also went to see a new obstetrician, my third try. Just like the other two I had seen, he stated that Asherman's only occurs when you stop menstruation completely and is extremely rare, occurring only after several D&C's. He encouraged me to "throw away the condoms" and assured me that most women with mild Asherman's have healthy pregnancies and are unaware of the scarring. I thought about all those women I'd just met in the online group who had paid for expensive, failed IVF procedures, underwent useless hormone treatments, and suffered successive miscarriages before they knew they had Asherman's. Even the best obstetricians want to believe that routine D&C's are completely harmless, and that any patient who suggests otherwise is just a "nut."

So I decided to trust the specialist rather than my obstetrician, and had the surgery under local anesthesia. He found scar tissue in the front of my uterus and removed it with microscissors. With my uterus on the video screen, I had intentionally taken my glasses off to blur my vision, instead focusing on breathing and relaxing. After the surgery, I had mild cramping and was given estrogen therapy and a balloon stent, which fills the uterus to prevent the sides from sticking together and re-scarring. Two periods later, another HSG X-ray came back clear, with the radiologist reporting an "unremarkable uterus." I laughed in ironic joy at the phrase, considering how truly remarkable it was to me. My ultrasound revealed an adequate seven-millimeter lining on cycle day twelve. I was given the green light to try to conceive again.

Three cycles later, I was pregnant. At close to seven weeks we saw a heartbeat. My husband and I were so very grateful for that moment: it was further than I'd ever gotten in a pregnancy. There was even a second empty sac, possibly a "vanishing twin," which made me even more grateful for the one heartbeat that we did see, considering what odds those little dividing cells were up against. Simply knowing that I was able to implant twice was a miracle and a testament to my surgeon's work.

But I soon learned that I was losing the pregnancy. A follow-up ultrasound at seven weeks showed no heartbeat. The day we learned of the loss, I was stunned to hear my obstetrician push another D&C on me because "my uterus had been fine all along." He cited "emotional closure" and "expediency," ignoring that my first D&C had offered quite the opposite. He went so far as to say that I might not be a near bathroom when the miscarriage came on—and tried to scare me with accounts of women passing "lemon-sized clots." But I waited ten days to see if the miscarriage would happen naturally, keeping my cell phone close at hand in case I needed to call my husband or the doctor, and actually aching for some physical pain just to numb my sorrow. But when I showed no signs of cramping, I resolved to take the drug misoprostol to expel the pregnancy at the advice of my Asherman's specialist. My new friend from the Asherman's support group had reported severe hemorrhaging from the drug: she had blacked out and needed to go to the emergency room via ambulance. So I packed a bag in case we needed to go to the ER and taped our doctor's phone numbers in bold letters on the bathroom mirror and the refrigerator. My husband laughed and said I was taping the numbers to "every vertical surface in the house." But then he realized how scared I really was. I sent him to the drug store to get the biggest maxi pads he could find and a bed liner normally used for incontinence.

About two weeks after fetal demise, I took painkillers and four misoprostol pills in the morning. Three and a half hours into it, with a heating pad and castor oil on my belly, I could feel the cramping and started light bleeding. The bleeding and pain became increasingly intense. Throughout the process, I drank a lot of fluids: pomegranate juice and coconut water to avoid getting light-headed. That evening, I passed a very large, palm-sized clot and felt immediate relief. I was left in a moment of existential awe. Unlike the D&C, the drugs allowed me the opportunity to mourn my pregnancy in a bodily way. I'm usually pretty squeamish, and have sometimes fainted during simple blood draws, but this ordeal gave me a new empathy for my physical body. Rather than resisting, I was remarkably calm, accepting what my body needed to do. Many women in my circumstance are even able to collect tissue for genetic testing. My specialist had told me not to worry about that, since it was highly unlikely that we could get answers from testing two weeks after fetal demise. But if I have another miscarriage, I now know I can methodically collect tissue to get answers about the loss.

On the third morning after taking the initial dose of pills, my obstetrician looked at the ultrasound image and said my uterus was clear and we could start trying to conceive again after one cycle. But about five weeks later, my basal temperatures were still pretty erratic. A woman in the Asherman's group had warned me to follow-up; only because of her did I go back to see my reproductive endocrinologist, who did a sonohysterogram (SHG), which revealed that the drugs had not evacuated everything. I had to have a second hysteroscopy with my Asherman's specialist for these "retained products of conception." According to my specialist, much of this tissue in my uterus had become fibrous over the last five weeks, making it more difficult to extract. Just before the surgery, I felt the familiar, debilitating regret: why hadn't I followed up sooner? In my attempt to heal from the loss and relax for a month, had I *again* prevented myself from ever having a child? I was under general anesthesia this time and it was a longer surgery than the first one. Again, I got the Cook stent (a balloon in the uterus to prevent scarring), this time for three weeks. I took antibiotics for that duration, and estrogen therapy for seven weeks.

I learned that sometimes there is no painless solution after a miscarriage, especially for those of us with a history of Asherman's. Natural, pharmaceutical, and surgical responses must be prescribed with the utmost care and thoughtfulness. I was still relieved to avoid the blind D&C: the drugs and the hysteroscopy were a much safer option for me. However, had the follow-up care after the use of misoprostol been more systemic, thorough and expedient, the surgery may have been easier and potentially less damaging to my uterus.

I won't ever know the cause of my most recent loss. I could not pursue genetic testing, and all blood testing for auto-immune infertility, another cause of recurrent miscarriage, are negative. There is a chance that some small area of scar tissue remained or re-formed in my uterus, causing the miscarriage. During an ultrasound, my reproductive endocrinologist noticed something that looked like scarring near the placenta, but she was not certain. Also, the fact that products of conception were so difficult to extract might indicate that the lining had not been totally intact before the loss. The early losses taught me to seek every answer, but this recent loss is teaching me to accept unknowns. Two and a half years into this journey, I can finally laugh and play with other women's babies again, releasing some of my own regret and sadness.

Uncertainty lingers. I've had a follow-up diagnostic hysteroscopy that showed a mostly normal uterus, but with one small area of irreparable damage. Though I was given the green light to try to conceive again, I am coming to terms with alternatives and being pragmatic. If I do get pregnant, I am at risk for various placental complications, or having an "incompetent" or weakened cervix caused by the repeated cervical dilations of my surgeries and procedures, which can lead to a second-trimester loss or premature delivery. I have my eyes wide open, having read accounts on the online Asherman's group of complications, tragedies, and successes. I will demand the right monitoring—if I am lucky enough to get there. I am reserving my emotional energy for what will be a long road ahead.

For many women with Asherman's, the psychological pain is triple-fold: first the devastating loss of a single pregnancy, then the incomprehensible threat of losing the chance at future pregnancies, and finally the almost complete devaluation of their experiences by their doctors. The greatest fault I find with the medical community is the simple lack of acknowledgment and information about Asherman's Syndrome. It is precisely at these moments when women are the most physically and emotionally vulnerable, unable to advocate for themselves—after a miscarriage, or the delivery of a baby—when doctors need to step up, show compassion, and take responsibility.

I reached a balance between Eastern and Western approaches to medicine, ultimately accepting the strengths and shortcomings of each system. I chose to accept surgery and use holistic treatments to support my healing. There have been many beneficial byproducts of the holistic treatments, and I plan to keep them up for the rest of my life. Many friends remark on a new glow: my skin is softer, and my hair shinier and fuller. I went from four prescriptions for seasonal allergies to only vitamins and an air purifier. Previously prone to flu and cold, I haven't been sick for the last two years. With Western medicine, we race against our biological clocks. And sometimes surely we must. But with holistic treatments, we at least have the feeling that we're slowing the clock and can keep it to a stroll.

And, perhaps most importantly, exploring Eastern medicine led me to trust my subjective bodily measures rather than simply listening to the "objective" voice of the doctor. Blindly trusting my doctor had burned me. So I reached another reconciliation: I had to balance my own vital but limited knowledge with that of several excellent and experienced practitioners, both doctors and acupuncturists. As I continue to struggle with Asherman's, the process of compiling this book, which values women's subjective accounts alongside doctors' studies, makes me feel less like a victimized sub-fertile woman and more like a compassionate and alive human being.

3. Doreen

To Her Uterus, Upon Travelling the Road to Asherman's Syndrome

Dear Uterus of Mine:

I didn't know. Words cannot begin to describe the sorrow I feel -- there is no adequate apology I can offer you.

I just didn't know. I think back on all those years of pain, all that blood; how old were we? 13, maybe - when it started? I had no idea. Mommy wasn't around and of course there was no one else I could have asked; there was no one I wanted to ask. I even remember being too embarrassed to ask Dad for money for pads. I just quietly and secretly dealt with it. Remember that brown printed towel I cut up to use instead?

I didn't know. I think of all the trains, buses, beds, couches, office chairs I soiled, in all the homes, places of employ, states and countries I've ever been. I remember joking to a female co-worker, "I can't be expected to know the velocity of my own body's fluids!" I laughed, I think. But it wasn't funny, was it? All the pain, all the blood. I'd neglected you; you were trying to tell me something - every month you tried - and every month I cavalierly thought, "At least I know everything's working!" And I would carry on, stashing as many pads as I could fit into my bag; stuffing an extra pair of pants in there, too. And all the while, I would read that having cramps and bleeding so heavily was indicative that something wasn't right - and I would dismiss it as being strange and hippie-like – a conspiracy theory.

I just didn't know. But finally, ironically, I was told by a man (!) of all people that what you were doing "wasn't normal." And it finally came to bear on me: all those years of pain, all that blood; all the "emergency" laundry loads, all the ruined underwear, clothes and bedding; the changing of pad after pad after pad after pad …

And then came the surgery - the one I thought would fix you, fix us. The one I thought would have brought us a baby by now. But when I woke up, they said it wasn't fibroids, as they'd thought; it was adenomyosis – in fact, they said that the entire back of you, my poor, dearest uterus, was one big adenomyoma – or tumor. They said you were one big tumor, basically, and it was hard to distinguish between you and it – the invasive, non-natural tissue. They took out what they could, but you would never be completely free of it. I thank the stars I knew to make sure no one took you away from me.

And then came the healing from that, and the waiting ... and then the sudden bleeding. They told me "it was nothing," that it was just a little cervicitis. They made me take a pregnancy test, to make sure. Of course it was negative: of course! But I was so full of hope, so open to the possibilities.

My periods - the ones that were supposed to be made lighter – were better for a little while. I finally experienced what most women know as "normal" periods. And so I started taking my basal body temperature every day, taking prenatal vitamins, adding supplements, swallowing herbs, drinking teas, adding tinctures – some to make my cervical mucus better, some to improve my overall fertility, some to make my ovulation "stronger." After a while, I could barely remember what I was taking everything for.

I didn't know. I didn't know that none of those things would be of any use to me. I never imagined, that day when I went for the HSG, that I would receive one of the most devastating pronouncements about you. I truly did believe that this was a routine check of my fallopian tubes and that it would all be fine. If my tubes were a little blocked, then the dye they inject (in order to get a view of you, my uterus, and everything connected with you) would do the job nicely and my tubes would be unblocked, as if by magic.

I had no idea, as I lay on that table, eagerly watching the screen –

excited to see what you would look like – that everything was about to change, yet again. It was painful when they injected the dye – like a searing chemical flame scorching my body from the inside. But all the while, my eyes never left that screen. And then there was silence: the doctor, the nurse both stopped talking; the jovial chit-chat came to an abrupt end. When I saw it, I didn't understand: "What am I looking at? Where is my uterus?" I asked. Still, silence. "Wait – is that it? That SPLOTCH?" They tried another balloon, to see if they could inflate me more, somehow, thinking they were missing something. Alas, no – they weren't missing anything: yes, the "splotch" was you, my uterus. You were not "open," let alone my fallopian tubes.

In the consult afterwards, the doctor uttered "gestational surrogate" and my world fell down around me. It would be at least a month before I could even speak the word "infertile," let alone do anything about it. And when I could finally say the word to myself, it seemed I couldn't stop saying it to myself: "I'm infertile. I'm infertile. I am infertile. Oh my god – I'm infertile."

It took a little more time before I realized that I still wanted to fight for you, dearest uterus. And then we embarked on a new road. First, we found someone who would say something other than "surrogate;" he is a reproductive endocrinologist, or "RE" -- someone who specializes in "infertility". In my heart, I thanked the gods for him as he, after reviewing all my records and performing a saline ultrasound, uttered the words, "Asherman's Syndrome". He then explained that he believed that surgery – the myomectomy – had caused you to scar. He said it wasn't insurmountable; that the scarring could be removed. He named a doctor about an hour's flight away, but I didn't quite hear him yet. I wanted to get home and digest it all – and to get online and do my own research about this syndrome.

Hundreds of dollars out of pocket and numerous tests had brought us to some hope. I would need to come up with a few thousand dollars, now, because the health insurance I have doesn't cover this. And I would need to travel. But in my research, I also found out that I was not alone: there are women all over the world with their own dear scarred uteruses. And they shared their empathy and knowledge with me and anyone like me ... we are all in the same boat. It was painful, though, to realize that not only were there women like me, there were women who had to travel further and pay more to get fixed, to heal, to finally conceive. This was not a comforting thought, but at least I knew that I wasn't the only one struggling against biology, against time, against finances – and most of all, against you, my dear uterus.

I talked to the doctor whose name the RE had mentioned. It turns out that this very doctor is considered an "A-list" specialist for the treatment – or surgical removal – of uterine scarring; he's an Asherman's guy. He told me my chances of success at pregnancy should I have the procedure (a hysteroscopy) done to remove the scarring inside you. He gave me some numbers; I don't remember them now, but they aren't good; they were better than zero, though, and he didn't say the words, "gestational surrogate." I said I would need to think about it, and that's what I'm doing now.

Can we do it, uterus? How will I pay for it? Who will help me when I'm pregnant? How will I raise him or her? How am I going to do all of this alone? What's the right thing to do? Should I just let it go? Should I just give up hope, give up my dream of becoming a mother? Or do I fight? Do I go on? Can I do it? Can I do it alone?

My dear uterus, I just don't know.

4. KAREN

When my husband and I got together, I knew that one of his "requirements" was that we would have our own child someday. He wants to be a father so bad. So, in May of 2008, I went to a new gynecologist to have my annual exam. I couldn't get into my regular gynecologist because he was booked until July of that year and my husband and I had began thinking of starting our family. My cycle had been non-existent since my regular gynecologist gave me a D&C approximately two years before, as a means to "restart" my cycle due to heavy, long periods.

My annual exam went well, nothing abnormal, but when we started talking to him about starting a family and my lack of periods, he became a bit worried. At first he put me on birth control to see if I would start a period...nothing. His second try was to put me on Provera for 10 days to try to force a period...nothing. As luck would have it, he was not only an excellent OB/GYN but his wife was doing her internship at the university in infertility so he mentioned something called Asherman's Syndrome and wanted to do a saline infused sonohistrogram (SIS) to see what might be going on in my uterus.

My husband and I went to the doctor's office that day very optimistic and excited about starting our family. When my new-found gynecologist tried to get the tube into my cervix to inject saline, he couldn't get it in. At this point, he sat us down and discussed with us that he believed it was most likely Asherman's Syndrome and he was just hoping that the cervix was the only thing that had scarred shut. This was the very beginning of a very long battle.

If I cannot get past this Asherman's Syndrome, my first fear is that my husband would leave me for someone that can give this to him. My second fear is that I would push him away thinking he SHOULD find someone that can give this to him. I know, and he has told me that even if we couldn't have children that we would continue with our lives and be happy, but one can't help but wonder.

At this time I searched for information on the Internet about Asherman's Syndrome and found Ashermans.org. There, I found many women that gave lots of suggestions and helpful information about what it was and the process to try to overcome it. I was advised by the very knowledgeable women to go straight to an "A-list" doctor (from the list of doctors on their site), who has had a lot of experience with Asherman's.

My gynecologist referred us to the university hospital's endocrinology department in which we were diagnosed with Asherman's Syndrome and we were told that my uterus appeared to be flat, like a pancake. We scheduled a surgery for that next week but the word surrogacy was mentioned, to which we politely advised them that we were not looking into that route yet.

When I was diagnosed with severe Asherman's Syndrome, we were informed that I – or my uterus -- was over 90% scarred. A hysteroscopy was performed and a Foley catheter was placed in my uterus to keep the walls from closing. I was prescribed a dose of estrogen to help the lining of my uterus grow (instead of scar tissue). They said that they had removed all the scar tissue, but I had to keep the catheter in for 10 days and come back to have it removed. This procedure was performed twice; each time my uterus was better but still scarring shut. After the third attempt, the university called and told us that they could no longer help us in our battle -- and that we needed to think about surrogacy or adoption.

It hurts my heart and breaks it into tiny pieces every time someone we know gets pregnant, I want to be happy for them but deep inside I just can't be. I see so many of my friends and family members go on to have their second or even third child and we are still fighting this, driving so many miles and spending so much money on just a hope that we might someday come home with a baby. We did give lots of thought to adoption and surrogacy, but we just don't have the money to fund such things.

This latest news was very devastating for us, but after one evening of crying our eyes out, we jumped into action to figure out our next steps. We found an "A-list doctor" about four and a half hours away from where we lived. After a phone call and emails I sent my files to him. He agreed to do the surgery and scheduled it for two weeks from that day.

This doctor's approach was similar but with a few extra twists. He performed the hysteroscopy and placed a Cook balloon stent in, which is in the shape of your uterus (makes sense, right?) that he left in for 30 days. He also gave me a higher dose of estrogen.

Again, this surgery made my uterus better but it still scarred once the balloon was removed. We moved on to weekly in-office hysteroscopic surgeries. I was given a local anesthetic and was awake while he removed scar tissue and could watch on the screen. This was a neat process, to see what it was supposed to look like, versus what my uterus actually did look like. The reason for the weekly procedures was to have minimum amount of trauma to the uterus while continuing to remove the new scar tissue that grew. This proved to be very profitable: we achieved a much higher success of keeping the scar tissue at bay.

During this process we decided to go through an IVF cycle, knowing that we would most likely need to freeze all my eggs, but we were fine with this and just wanted to be prepared when my uterus was ready. We did this while still doing the multiple in-office hysteroscopies to make sure I did not scar further during IVF.

It has been very hard for us to try to explain to every doctor, friend or family member why it is so important for us to have a child. Early in our diagnosis, the university doctors could not understand why we did not want to entertain the idea of surrogacy or adoption. It is important for everyone to know that we are not against those options, and we have actually made plans in case this is a route that we need to take. We believe that Asherman's is not something the healthcare system recognizes a treatable; it seems they think that it is something that we should just accept and resign ourselves to. But Asherman's *can* and has been treated: you just have to find someone willing to invest in you.

But I feel like Asherman's Syndrome has started to control my life with doctor appointments, what I can eat, can't eat, medicine I take, money I can or can't spend and how my marriage will play out. Nothing is in my control any longer. My life has been taken from me by this awful disease and I want to do is get it back, but there is no cure, no one treatment that will work for everyone. I ask myself all the time, "When will it be too much? When will we just give up and try to move on with this void in our lives?" I want to tell the whole world that a D&C is dangerous and no one should ever have one, although I know that there are some that are in need of such a procedure. It is a fight every day, emotionally, to watch as your friends and relatives move on and have their families while you are stuck holding on to hope.

But if hope is all we have, then hope is what we will hold on to. To date, we have performed three surgeries with the A-list doctor and two at the university and too many in-office hysteroscopies to count. My uterus is approximately 60% open with sporadic lining ranging from 2 mm to 4.58 mm, which is quite a feat from the original diagnosis of 90% scarring. Our current plan of action is 4 mg of estrogen orally, 4mg estrogen vaginally and

2 ml of estrogen injection. We are looking to get a decent lining and trying to transfer some of our frozen embryos. If this doesn't work, our wonderful A-list doctor has vowed that he will continue to try as long as we are willing to put the time in. We are determined to have a child and believe that we will be one of the many success stories to come.

5. RHONDA

When my husband and I decided we were ready to start our family, we went about this new stage in our life with a relaxed approach. We decided to stop using oral contraceptives and just see what would happen. I did not pay any attention to my cycle. We just looked at it as though we were not necessarily "trying" to conceive; instead, we were simply not avoiding pregnancy anymore. We felt we had time and that this was a healthy approach. I did not want to try to plan the perfect timeline for pregnancy and delivery - I always felt in my heart that it would happen when it was time.

To our surprise, we conceived in August 2008, only five months after I stopped taking the pill. We were over the moon! I will never forget the day I found out. I didn't sleep at all that night. I was too excited. The dream of our family becoming a reality was overwhelming. There was suddenly so much to think about, so much to do, and so many people to tell.

Everything seemed to be going along well. My belly was growing and I had all the right symptoms. I actually felt pretty good for the most part. My obstetrician wanted to hold off until twelve weeks for my first ultrasound. I was disappointed, but since everything seemed to be okay and as this was my first pregnancy, I trusted that this was standard.

Early in October, at eleven weeks, I began spotting. I wasn't alarmed at first since I knew that this could be normal. On the third day of spotting with no signs of letting up, I was concerned. It was a Sunday. I asked my husband to take me to the emergency room to get checked out. After much poking and prodding and what felt like an eternity, the doctor told us that cardiac activity could not be detected. The room went dark and I wept uncontrollably. The doctors and nurses didn't come right out and say what had happened. We received no details. The doctor instructed us to come to his office the following day for a follow-up ultrasound before proceeding, just to be sure. I was in denial. I knew deep down inside what had happened, but the medical staff left plenty of room for false hopes with their vagueness. My mind began to race: "What if…?"; "Maybe it was just the ultrasound machine they used…"; "This is all just a big scare." I felt like I had been completely blindsided.

The next day at the doctor's office, we were told that we had a "missed miscarriage." The fetal pole had measured only about seven weeks, but I was eleven and a half weeks along. How could this be? I still felt pregnant. My body was still responding to the pregnancy. Why didn't I get an ultrasound when I requested it at my eight-week appointment? I would have known something was wrong weeks ago. Why is this happening? How could I not know? I felt so foolish. I sobbed uncontrollably. I was numb. I felt as though the room was spinning. All these happy women filled the waiting room, with their healthy pregnant bellies and beautiful newborn babies.

The doctor called us back in to discuss my options, which seemed simple. I could do "expectant management" (closely monitoring and waiting for the miscarriage to expel naturally) or I could have a dilation and curettage (D&C). He explained the benefits of the D&C. His explanation sounded reasonable and attractive. He told us that we would have emotional closure and that this would enable us to move on quicker in order to try again, and that there was a lower risk for infection this way. He assured us it was low risk. Being in a complete fog, and trusting his expertise, I followed his advice and opted for the D&C. We scheduled it for the following day. Not having ever been in the hospital or having had any type of surgery, I was scared. Grief was settling in as the reality of my hopes and dreams was simultaneously crushed.

Fast forward to post-D&C. I eagerly awaited the return of my monthly cycle, as others said to me, "Just relax, it will come and you will get pregnant again in a few months." From what I had researched, I knew I could expect my period within four to six weeks after the D&C. I kept in touch with my gynecologist's office as I waited and waited. They kept telling me to be patient and not to worry. I took progesterone for ten days. Nothing happened. On December 31, 2008, at twelve weeks post-D&C, my doctor met with me in his office. After an internal ultrasound, he told me that my lining was very thin and that it was likely stress that was causing the delay in the return of my cycle. He told me I could "win an Oscar for anxiety," which only increased the guilt I felt. Was I the cause of this? How could I possibly "calm down" and not feel stressed? What did it mean that my lining was thin? I hadn't had so much as a sign of spotting. I had only experienced cyclic cramping episodes that were enough to keep me in bed the entire day, feeling miserable with pain. The doctor ordered blood tests and concluded that if they came back okay (which they did), we would be patient and wait for my cycle to return until four months post D&C. If still no period, he would put me back on birth control to start my cycle. His plan did not sit well with me. I left his office crying and feeling hopeless. He had completely discounted my situation and made me feel I was the cause. He hadn't even suggested looking further into it. I knew deep down inside something was not right. That was the last time I saw him.

I immediately began searching for a second opinion. I received a referral from a friend to a local fertility specialist and immediately booked an appointment for February 2009. After a consultation and internal ultrasound, the reproductive endocrinologist suspected Asherman's Syndrome. He explained his plan, which was to put me on estrogen immediately to begin building my lining. Then, once the lining was a little suppler, he would do a hysterosalpingogram (HSG) to officially diagnose my condition, and schedule a hysteroscopy to remove the scarring. He explained that I would need to be patient.

Soon after this appointment, I found the Asherman's Syndrome online support group through Yahoo! Groups. I did not realize at the time how valuable this group would be, and just how blessed I was to have stumbled across it. I had no idea what was in store for me.

I began researching and learning more about Asherman's Syndrome through my new group. It was very overwhelming but the more I learned, the more empowered I felt.

I had my HSG in April, which concluded a moderate case of approximately 40-50% scarring with adhesions in the uterus and one fallopian tube blocked. My surgery was May 29th, 2009. I ended up having a laparoscopy with the hysteroscopy, concluding about 60% intrauterine scarring and adhesions with one blocked tube. I also had some mild scarring over my cervix.

The surgery was successful. My uterus looked great and my tube was open. A balloon was placed to prevent the uterine walls from re-adhering. I had an appointment three days post-op to remove the balloon. Boy, was I glad to get that dreadful thing out! I had a tough time recovering the first few days, but within a couple of weeks I was feeling much better. My energy was slow to return, but with each day I was stronger. The doctor ordered me to continue the estrogen for a couple more months, and then we would meet for a follow-up.

My first period since my pregnancy arrived, right on cue, just four weeks after surgery. I was thrilled beyond words! This was a huge milestone and gave me reassurance that everything was back on track.

In August 2009, it had been two months since the surgery and I was eager to have my follow-up appointment. I was hoping the doctor would say my lining looked good and take me off the estrogen. I had been on it for a total of six months and I was more than ready. I had two perfect periods, right on target with the calendar. I was pretty sure I had ovulated both cycles as well. To my surprise, after an internal ultrasound, the doctor said that I could stop taking the estrogen and that we could start trying to conceive. I nearly fainted right there in his office! I was overcome by emotion, hope and excitement. Knowing how eager my husband and I were to get another chance at conception, the doctor talked to me about follicular stimulation and intrauterine insemination (IUI). I explained that we wanted to try to conceive on our own for a few months.

In October 2009, after much thought and at the difficult milestone of one year since losing our baby, I gained the courage to write a letter to the doctor that gave me Asherman's Syndrome. My newfound focus was to help spread the word about this condition and promote awareness through education. Asherman's Syndrome is more common than the obstetric community believes; I felt compelled to notify this doctor of what has transpired as a result of the D&C he performed on me just one year earlier. In that one year, I had acquired thousands of dollars worth of medical bill debt, not to mention the emotional strain and stress that accompanied this journey. This process was all-consuming and it was immensely important for me to make him aware. My hope was, and still is, to save other women from this grief. There is strength and power in knowledge.

It is the beginning of a new year, 2010, that I write this story ... my story. I just turned 35 years old. Trying to conceive has been a rollercoaster. Hope is lost and regained time and time again. I second guess myself and every decision I make. I change my mind every time I think about our plan. I have put countless Plan As and Plan Bs into place. I no sooner get one issue settled in my mind, finding a solution, than another unsettling issue pops up. This has not been an easy road, and I have not even battled the journey as long as others. I do believe my happy ending will come, even if it is not the ending I hoped for and planned on. I give it all to God. I know He has a plan for us, and I know I can only control so much. This is what keeps me going.

Looking back, I wish I had known the real risks involved with a D&C following a missed miscarriage. I wish I had known that 30% of women who have a missed miscarriage that results in a D&C end up with Asherman's Syndrome. I had never even heard of Asherman's Syndrome until I was diagnosed. Clearly my doctor did not know about it either, which is frightening. I also wish I would have followed my instincts and demanded the ultrasound at my eight-week appointment. I was told it was too soon and did not know to object the time.

As you read these stories of sorrow, struggle, strength, hope and gratitude, I hope you will remember a couple of important things. Always be your own advocate. Do not trust anyone but yourself. Follow your instincts and your heart ... and most importantly, keep fighting! The women I have come to know and befriend on the Asherman's Syndrome online support group have helped me through some of the darkest times in my life, when no one else understood. They have taught me so much, and I am forever grateful.

II. POST ASHERMAN'S PREGNANCY AND CHILDBIRTH

6. CHRISTY

My post-Asherman's baby arrived on August 28, 2008 with no complications. Her name is Reese Sheri Brunton and she was born at 37 weeks 4 days weighing 6 lbs. 2 ounces. Hopefully my story will give hope to other women who are starting this journey.

After a Caesarean section to deliver my twin girls in May 2005, I needed a D&C (dilation and curettage) because I had retained placenta from a hemorrhage that occurred two weeks after delivery. This is when my battle with Asherman's Syndrome started. After my twin girls were born, I did not have a period for nine months so went to see my obstetrician for a consultation. This doctor, (not the OB who caused this) mentioned the word "Asherman's." I wanted to know more so within 24 hours I found the Asherman's Syndrome website and had essentially diagnosed myself.

As suggested on the site, I found an A-List doctor, met with him to discuss my condition and then had my first surgery in February 2007. I found out that I was 100% scarred (called a complete whiteout). He was able to get 80% of the scar tissue out at the first surgery.

I had a second surgery in May 2007 but had trouble with the stent falling out so I ended up re-scarring. I had a third and final surgery in August 2007 and my hysterosalpingogram (HSG) came back showing only 10% scarring. After that, my doctor gave me the green light to try conceiving in October.

For two months, my husband and I tried to get pregnant. In December 2007, I had my endometrial lining measured at mid-cycle and it came back at 4 mm. With such a thin lining, I knew it wasn't going to be our month but Mother Nature had another idea. Somehow I was pregnant! My AS doctor started me on progesterone right away and watched me closely during the first trimester.

I am happy to say that I had a typical, uncomplicated pregnancy. I bled only one night at eight weeks and had some nausea due to the progesterone in the first three months. I was being watched closely by a high risk doctor. I received what seemed like a million ultrasounds (in reality, more like 25) but everything looked good. I did start having some low amniotic fluid issues around week 36 but I don't believe these were due to my AS. I delivered at 37.5 weeks via Caesarean section. We were prepared in the operating room for a hysterectomy just in case since I was showing some signs of possible placenta accreta, but I ended up not having to have a hysterectomy even though my placenta was a little sticky.

So, all in all, a great post-AS pregnancy. I still can't believe I have my baby girl after 100% scarring and three surgeries hundreds of miles from home! Most doctors would have written me off and told me to adopt, but Dr. Charles March, the doctor I found through the Asherman's support network was able to give me my baby!

Good luck to all of you starting your journey … there are many happy endings now that you know what you are dealing with!

7. LUCILA

I was thirty-five and living in Australia when we found out we were expecting twins. My partner and I felt so lucky that we might have an instant family! But sadly, at seventeen weeks pregnant we discovered the babies had a severe case of "Twin to Twin Transfusion Syndrome," a very rare disease that affects identical twins. After much deliberation, we decided to terminate the pregnancy. We decided to induce so that we could have a chance to say goodbye to our boys. They were born at 8:00pm on the 5th January 2002.

Despite being considered a high-risk pregnancy (because I was expecting twins), I had never seen the Consultant[1] of the Hospital for any of my pregnancy appointments. One of his Registrars handled the delivery of the twins. After the delivery the placenta remained and the injection I was given to expel it didn't work. Early the next morning the Registrar explained to me that we had waited long enough and I needed to have a manual D&C. A surgery that was supposed to take twenty minutes took more than one hour. During the surgery the placenta got stuck and broke into little pieces that she had to remove one by one, aided by an ultrasound machine. Afterwards, I was given antibiotics and a midwife came to my house for five days to check on me. I had a slight fever but she said it was due to the fact that my breasts were full of milk and I was obviously not breastfeeding. No one suspected an infection.

The midwife delivered lots of written information about what to expect after such a loss. The leaflets mentioned that a bloody discharge was normal for some time, but quantity or duration of the discharge were not

---

[1] In Australia, a Consultant is a senior medical doctor in a hospital. In university-hospitals a Consultant will usually supervise a number of Registrars. A Registrar is a medical doctor receiving advanced training.

specific And I had no "bad odor" that the leaflets said would signal an infection. Since I had no previous experience to compare with, I thought that the bleeding must be normal. I was a Brazilian in a foreign country with no family members around and only a limited network of friends to compare postpartum experiences with.

Few days later, I started to get really tired with mild crampy pain. I remember I could not walk more than a block and lacked energy for doing anything around the house. Over the next two weeks, the pain continued to worsen and I passed a clot that was the size of an olive. My GP (General Practitioner) ordered an ultrasound and when the Radiologist looked at my uterus she told me to go straight to the hospital. She phoned my GP who concurred. I had an infection and my uterus was full of blood. There were no beds available at the hospital but I finally got to speak on the phone with the Consultant responsible for my case. This was the first time we spoke since my pregnancy. He seemed casual, asking whether I preferred to be admitted to the emergency room and wait for a bed or come back another day. By this stage I was extremely tired, it felt hard even to simply stand there holding the phone at the hospital's reception. I was in pain and scared. I had had enough. I said to him: "I am not a doctor, I don't know how bad my case is, perhaps if you came to meet me at the reception you could see the ultrasound report and photos, and maybe analyze my situation. I can only tell you that the Radiologist after looking at my uterus said I should come straight to the hospital, and I think she was extremely concerned."

The Consultant did come to see me in the waiting room, looked at the Radiologist's report, and stated the same options: admission in the emergency room, stay for the night and have a surgery (D&C) the next morning with another one of his Registrars; or go home, wait for two days and come back as a day patient, when he would then perform the surgery himself. I imagined as a Consultant he would be more experienced, so I went home and waited. The procedure was called a guided D&C, as he also used an ultrasound machine. After the surgery he said I was fine, and I should expect my period in six weeks´ time.

Well, this period did not come. Sometime after the first or the second surgery, I developed Asherman's and I was never warned of this possible outcome. Six weeks later I went back to my GP and told her I still had no period but an increased amount of a jelly-like discharge and I was worried something was wrong. She said the sadness of my loss had probably caused the lack of menstruation. I went to see this GP in February, March and April and got the same diagnosis every time. She would check my hormone levels, talk to me about losing the babies and say that my period would probably come next month. In my last consultation with her I said: "Are you SURE there is nothing that could have gone wrong in the D&Cs? There is nothing that could have damaged my uterus?" It seemed a statement of basic common sense but she then kept on saying that the causes were emotional. Finally she agreed to talk to a gynecologist about my case. Two days later, she called with a referral to a gynecologist. She had spoken to a doctor who mentioned I could have developed some adhesions. She said this condition was extremely rare but the gynecologist wanted to check it out. That day I researched the Internet on uterine adhesions and D&Cs and I found the Asherman's site. I was amazed how similar my story was to so many other women from around the world. I discovered a new meaning for the world "rare". I had been told it was rare to get pregnant with twins, rare to have identical twins, rare to have TTTS, and rare to have Asherman's. I had all of the above.

Looking back, I can see how the hospital system and doctors provided me with very poor quality care. Although the Registrar used the ultrasound machine to check my uterus during the surgery and prescribed antibiotics, I still developed what they call a "hidden" infection and Asherman's because of remaining products of conception. At the time, we were so distressed with the experience of losing our babies that we couldn't really assess the situation. We were in 'survival mode' – waking up in the morning to wait for the evening to arrive. Life had come to a standstill and nothing mattered. Today I find it more than a bit bizarre that you have to insist that the doctor in charge of your case comes to see you at the reception desk of a hospital. And because of our experience of grief and loss, the GP simply dismissed me as depressed instead of trying to investigate possible causes for my lack of period.

But I still went to the same hospital for my diagnostic hysteroscopy. On the day of the hysteroscopy the gynecologist recommended by my GP who was supposed to perform my surgery didn't show up. Apparently he had an emergency call at the last minute. At the entrance of the theatre, I was introduced to his Registrar. I cried and said I was not having the surgery. I was so scared of having mistakes in my uterus again. I didn't want a Registrar to perform my surgery; I wanted a proper doctor, a very experienced doctor. I felt so tired and hopeless and thought people were just mistreating me. In the end, I did have the surgery with the Registrar under the condition that she would just look at my uterus and not attempt to do anything else during the surgery. And so she gave me little pictures of my uterus full of adhesions and the Asherman's diagnosis.

After the surgery I finally realized we needed a change. We changed doctors and hospitals. Through the Asherman's site I found information about the syndrome and its treatment. I read and read and read. Somehow I decided that our life was not going to be taken over by this sad story. I started to analyze all the anger I was feeling towards figuring out what I needed to know and do in order to overcome Asherman's. I decided to take matters in my own hands and use what had happen to me as a lesson: to me and to everyone that was around us. I downloaded medical articles about Asherman's. I tried to learn as much as I could about it. I contacted a new doctor who was recommended by a German Asherman's specialist. I sent him an email explaining my story and he was so kind in his reply. I went back to see my GP, since I needed a letter of referral to see the specialist I wanted. I gave her lots of printed Asherman's information and the address of the Asherman's website.

In my first visit with the Asherman's specialist, I brought a little notebook with lots of questions. I made sure his treatment was close to what I had read was the best treatment for Asherman's cases. The doctor explained the syndrome, drew pictures of my uterus, did an ultrasound of my uterus, talked about the treatment and said I was not the worst case he had seen. Later, I was diagnosed with moderate Asherman's; my adhesions were at the lower part of my cavity and my cervix was blocked. The treatment would be long and involved probably more than one surgery. He said in his experience somewhere between one and six surgeries, with an average three surgeries. He prescribed some estrogen. When we left his consulting room I was happy and convinced I would finally get good treatment. It was not only the fact that he knew about Asherman's, but that he was knowledgeable enough to explain to us about it in simple words. It felt like we were in a partnership and we three (the doctor, my partner and I) would do all that we could to overcome this situation.

My first operative hysteroscopy was in July 2002. The surgery lasted only five minutes because my Asherman's specialist perforated my uterus. The surgery is very delicate because the doctor can't see where he has to go. Well, he went in the wrong direction and reached the walls of my cavity.

When I woke up from the surgery I saw that my partner had been crying. He didn't know how to tell me that the surgery went wrong. I thought I was very unlucky but I remembered I had read on the Asherman's website that perforation sometimes happens even with the best specialists. I was told I needed to wait for three months before having another surgery so that the walls of my cavity would heal. I did indeed need a break and I went on holidays to see my family.

My second surgery was in October 2002. This surgery was successful: the doctor was able to clean my uterus from the adhesions. Unfortunately, the adhesions reformed at my cervix. I stopped with the estrogen hormones in November as my doctor said the lining in my cavity was good: 7 mm. I had two more surgeries in November and December 2002, but each time adhesions reformed at my cervix. The doctor said that at each surgery the amount of adhesions in my cervix was less and less, nevertheless adhesions were still there. In January 2003 I had my fifth and final surgery. This time the doctor used a barrier, a spray gel, to prevent adhesions from reforming.

In January 2003, after fifteen months of no period, I finally got a period five days after the surgery. I was so happy and grateful that I was bleeding again. It was an amazing feeling. I looked back on those days when I used to complain about having my periods and moods and all that comes with it. Once I didn't have my period anymore, I just felt so miserable. When it came back it was such a RELIEF. My second period was not as good as the first one, I was one week late, and it was much darker blood and less quantity, but still it was a period, so I was definitely happy. In fact, I think part of me was just fully determined to be positive, to put grief and sorrow behind us. I did not want to fret over the meaning of 'dark blood' I just held the fact that 'there was blood'.

I never got a third period because I got pregnant. I could not believe how lucky we were. We were given a second chance to have a family. But I knew that pregnancy after Asherman's was not easy. There are so many things that can go wrong, like incompetent cervix or problems with the placenta and therefore with the baby's development. It was very scary, but I tried to control my anxiety by reading a lot about all the possible outcomes. When I was six weeks pregnant I started to notice a few dark blood spots, but they were so little and very seldom. I thought the uterus was expanding and imagined that could cause the release of some old blood trapped somewhere. However, at nine weeks, I was happily shopping for a birthday present when I felt something weird coming down my pants. I went to the toilet and to my horror I saw a heavier full on, very red blood coming. I took a cab home and phoned my partner in despair. He took me to the office of my Asherman's specialist, where his partner performed an ultrasound and checked my uterus. He found the heartbeat of my little baby. It was the best sound I have ever heard. I went home and was literally lying down for most of the next two weeks.

At this time we left Australia for New Zealand so I asked my Asherman's specialist for a referral to an obstetrician in New Zealand. I had great care this time with an entire group of specialists looking after my pregnancy. I also continued to correspond with my Asherman's specialist in Australia and would consult him via email about questions regarding post Asherman's pregnancy. He was amazingly supportive, always answering my questions and emails promptly. I sent several updates to him and his partner, even when there was nothing really going wrong. I just wanted them to learn from my case, as a post-Asherman's patient, so they could use this information to treat other women in the future.

During the pregnancy I had many ultrasounds. I had weekly visits at the clinic to check the baby. The amount of surgeries I had --seven in one year!-- meant that I was more susceptible to developing problems with my cervix. Thus, we decided to go for a preventative cerclage. I had read of too many cases of incompetent cervix and second trimester losses in post Asherman's pregnancies and I didn't want to risk losing another baby. The cerclage also had some risks, but we decided to have the procedure because I felt I would be more relaxed. It was put in place at fifteen weeks. I had no infections from the procedure and from then on my pregnancy was perfect. I was of course still very anxious. I was advised to avoid too much exercise and to stay near a hospital. At thirty-seven weeks the baby was breech so we decided for an elective Caesarean. In my appointment the day before the surgery, the ultrasound showed the baby had turned. Even so, my partner and I along with the doctors decided for the C-section. My baby was born in November 2003 at thirty-eight weeks. I had two doctors attending the surgery and fortunately there were no complications. My little boy was perfect, the placenta detached from the walls in one piece this time. My partner and I were so happy and relieved. It was the best day of my life.

Losing the twin babies and then getting Asherman's was such an extreme ordeal for my partner and me. Nevertheless, it made our relationship stronger and today I feel I am a much better person. As a couple, we managed to survive through the worst of times and we learned we could definitely count on one another. We know we can stand each other's pain and feelings of hopelessness. There is no one in this world that loved our twin babies as much as my partner and I. There is no one in this world that knows the intensity of the frustration we experienced. How unfair it felt that we were deprived of grieving for our loss, because we needed to learn about Asherman's. But together we learned and found the answers, the treatment and the support we needed. I am a stronger woman: I listen to my body, I trust in my feelings whenever I think something is wrong and I ask questions and demand what I want and deserve from doctors.

I now have regular periods, but they are fairly light. I never felt I was "ready" to get pregnant again, to go through that whole experience again. Despite being a little family, we are a very happy one. Our son has just turned 6 years old and he is the happiest little man on this planet. He is so special in so many different ways. I look at him every day and he instantly warms my heart up. He always makes me think about how lucky we actually are.

8. CORINNA

THE POWER OF ONLINE SUPPORT GROUPS

This is an article on how we empowered women from all over the world to regain their fertility and how numerous strongly desired babies were born despite the doctors´ inability to help with their mothers' infertility. It is an article about the power of support groups, specifically online support groups, which are able to gather hundreds of patients with a supposedly rare syndrome in a very short period of time, simply because of a new technology of communication. And it is also a story of a strong-minded lady, the founder of the Asherman´s Syndrome support group and how online friendships can become quite real.

When I joined the International Asherman´s Association back in 2000, I was member no. 48 and there were over 3000 members´ messages in the archive at the online communication platform. It took me roughly ten nights - and a husband, who thought I was nuts - to read all of them and to finally find great information on the syndrome which I suffered from. I had just had my first operation for Asherman´s Syndrome with an expert (I didn´t know of his expertise when joining the group and felt a huge relief when I later learned that he was one of a few worldwide to treat severe Asherman's). After one and a half years of major questions, setbacks, incorrect D&Cs, useless hormonal therapies and above all a huge feeling of frustration in regards to my sudden and out of control infertility (after the birth of my first daughter and retained placenta), ten nights seemed little investment. The emotional gain of being able to talk to 47 other women with similar problems was invaluable and kept my head above the water.

I had been directed to the support group by a woman I had "talked to" online in a general fertility discussion forum. I will be forever grateful to this lady who had been so kind to offer this life changing advice to me - a virtual stranger from the great World Wide Web. She also helped me find a German expert by giving me the name of an American hysteroscopist who had originally been trained in Germany. I ended up taking the train 450 kilometers to the recommended German doctor, talked to him personally for one hour and was rewarded by his opinion, that the other German hysteroscopist, who had just done my surgery, was one of the best worldwide to do so. My personal Asherman´s Syndrome journey got fair wind, and to cut a long story of one more diagnostic hysteroscopy, divorce and new partnership short, I was pregnant by March 2001 with my longed for baby no. 2 who was born via C-section nearly nine months later.

But my personal life had not only been affected positively in regards to my fertility, I also started to meet many wonderful ladies online. I was able to share my anxiety during this and the following pregnancies; I got precious advice, both psychologically and physically; Women listened to me and I listened to them. And I was able to share my knowledge about Asherman´s Syndrome. A great collection of medical articles about this syndrome was compiled and as patients we compared our medical stories with a data spreadsheet (which later served as the basis for scientific research). We rated different doctors with carefully considered criteria (i.e. A-lister, B-lister) and in 2006 and 2011 we organized shuttle conferences in San Francisco and Las Vegas for all hysteroscopists with expertise on Asherman´s Syndrome to meet and exchange their experiences. We also organized the first International Conference on the Treatment of Asherman´s Syndrome in Hamburg, Germany, in 2013 including four live surgeries. We published a DVD on state of the art Asherman´s treatment with live surgery videos from this conference[2]. I held speeches about the empowerment of patients through online support groups, and a friend of mine wrote her PhD about the positive effect of the support group membership on the patient´s treatment outcome[3]. We founded the International Asherman´s Association in the USA with its Board of Directors meeting almost every month to continue numerous efforts on getting the word out on Asherman´s. In other words: together with the pioneers on minimal invasive gynecology surgery worldwide we became the real experts on this condition. My active medical English vocabulary grew immensely, so did the amount of hours I spent at the computer.

But above all I had the privilege to meet the founder of the Asherman´s Syndrome Support Group personally, when Poly came to have surgery with the expert here in Germany. At the time I was living in an apartment with only one bedroom. I apologetically told Poly and suggested a nearby hotel for her stay, but to my surprise she asked me to be able to stay in my apartment in order not to be alone. My new partner and I picked her up from the airport on a cold winter morning, I drove with her to the clinic, waited for her surgery and her recovery and drove her back in my car. I felt so sorry when she was sick, stopped the car twice on the motorway and tried to do anything to comfort her then and during the following days. It was my humble way of showing my appreciation for what she had done for me and other ladies when she founded the group and gave so generously a lot of her time in running it. Poly and I spent the next four days together, never separated, with lots of laughter, honest thoughts and lots of mutual interests.

---

[2] Available with German and English presentations upon request, mail to cm.dartenne@web.de.
[3] Klemm, Christine 2007, http://www.asherman.de/fileadmin/downloads/diss-klemm.pdf (German)

Since then Poly has been an inspiring and very special person to my family and me.

After my second baby had been born in December 2001, she kindly accepted to be my daughter's Godmother.

Poly's visit here to have surgery with one of the leading experts in the field started my series of personal experiences with other ladies from all over the world. I decided to assist other women get the excellent medical treatment I had received, no matter from which country they would come. During their stay for treatment at the clinic I translated for them, I helped with travel arrangements and I stayed in mail contact with them after their stay here.

There are numerous memories of exceptional social encounters: One of the first patients to stay with my family and me was Jane from Kenya. She arrived with her husband, a biologist with research interest in frogs. Her rich dark skin contrasted greatly with my baby's pale milky skin, so that I can immediately visualize the photo we took with the two cheek to cheek. At her second visit here in Germany, she brought with her the most delicious African spices.

Nathalie, a French woman living in the States, overwhelmed my children with top label clothes I could never have afforded myself.

Dawn from England held my third newly born tiny baby when the baby had just been discharged from the hospital's Neonatal Intensive Care Unit. She held her so cautiously and was reminded once more why she wanted to get help with her scarred uterus.

Ana from Spain arrived with her husband Tony and her son David, who instantly started playing with my first daughter, Lea, without a bit of German. Years later they offered Lea to stay with them in Spain to improve her Spanish.

Ivana from Italy had surgery at the clinic when a TV team filmed a documentary on the clinic´s work. They filmed my tears when the doctor informed her that her uterine status sadly was beyond repair. It was then and there that I had to accept that Asherman´s Syndrome does not only lead to a happy ending, despite every possible effort.

Then there was Pilar from Spain, who arrived at the clinic without me knowing. She spoke neither German nor English. Ana, then moderator of the Spanish Asherman´s Syndrome support group, rang me immediately and asked me to help Pilar. I had a hard time persuading the clinic to operate on her regardless, given that she would otherwise have spent a lot of money in vain. The clinic finally agreed when a friend of mine translated the necessary information by phone.

I met Jacqueline from Berlin who I visited in the hotel where she was recovering from her surgery. There I suddenly started suffering from a stomach virus and her partner gentlemanlike offered to drive me home (60 kilometers away!) and take the train back to the hotel. A year and many phone calls and private visits later she asked me to be her maid of honor at their wedding. We are still in contact regularly.

Nina and her husband from Finland have remained friends ever since they came to Hamburg to have the first AS surgery. Nina is my fourth daughter´s Godmother and every year we fly over to Helsinki to see her and her family.

Both Helena and Louiza from the UK were early members of the support group with AS stories resembling mine. They had surgery in Hamburg, gave birth to their post AS child and later helped us tremendously when we needed to travel to the UK for a special therapy for my second daughter. Once they came for medical help to Germany, now each year my daughter and I travel for medical help to the UK. Experts are out there and other patients (via online support groups) are willing to go out of their way to help us find them.

The more women I accompanied to the clinic, the more competent support I felt I could give. Since 2001, hundreds of women from all over Europe, from Africa, from the Middle East, even from the U.S.A. (surgery here is much cheaper) have travelled to have their uterine scarring removed, gently and with the best possible instruments, so they could hope to carry a child again. I can only guess how much courage it takes to come to a foreign country to have surgery there without speaking the country´s language. Meeting these brave ladies was always an intense and fruitful encounter. Not only did I learn about many more personal and medical aspects on Asherman´s Syndrome, I also learned about different cultures, i.e. the meaning of lost fertility in other cultures. I listened to a woman from Africa talking about her fear of being shunned by her family for her inability to bear a child.

Since I shared times of hope and joy, but also doubt and despair with these patients, many of these relationships formed into private friendships. The most rewarding moments throughout this volunteer work though have been the ones when I opened a letter and discovered another birth announcement card from a former Asherman´s Syndrome patient. Like me, most of these women had been told they could never carry another child. And yet, with the help of the online support group, Poly´s determined work to spread the word about this syndrome and, of course, the excellent medical treatment they received here, they had another chance to become pregnant and hold a baby in their arms. A few of these women weren´t so fortunate and even with surgery from the expert here in Germany nothing could be done to repair their loss of fertility. I grieved with them at the time and I rejoiced with them years later when they told me about adoption, wonderful step-children or other meaningful ways to go on with their life.

In 2004 and 2006 I gave birth to my third and fourth child, two more daughters. My own medical ordeal found a happy ending. I am the mother of four girls, a dream I always had, a dream that was left hanging on a perilous thread, waiting to be shattered by unexperienced doctors who not only had overseen remaining placenta pieces from my original delivery, but also did not feel obliged to further investigate after my original diagnosis of severe Asherman´s Syndrome.

Like the other members (more than a thousand members so far), with the help of the support group I learned to demand better medical care despite this syndrome being a rare one. I learned to take my own health into my hands and discuss it with the doctor, as a team, becoming involved in the decision making process.

As already mentioned, a friend of mine wrote her dissertation on the relevance of online support groups of rare diseases. With Poly´s and my help she conducted a questionnaire survey in the Asherman´s Syndrome support group. Her results clearly reflect our experiences: The membership in the Asherman´s Syndrome support group significantly helped the members to gain better medical treatment in a shorter period of time.

I personally consider online support groups a revolution. With the help of the International Asherman´s Syndrome support group babies were allowed to come into this world, because their mothers (and even fathers) were not only given new hope, but at the same time they were given substantial information for further steps to take. They were armed with questions for their doctors and were made aware of answers which should prick their ears. All of this was and is a matter of emails reaching the members in seconds, there are no national or social boundaries, and all of it is accessible for just a very small donation to the IAA. The online relationships are based on mutuality. A problem shared is indeed a problem halved and even a problem solved, especially when it comes to sharing profound knowledge and experience.

Asherman´s Syndrome is a condition written about more than 100 years ago, but it took 90 years to become a condition, which at last is talked about and finally recognized among the medical professionals. Poly founded the support group in December 1999, nearly three decades ago. Her dedication in addition to the new communication technology has made a huge difference for more than a thousand women and their families. It has made a huge difference in my life. It has worked wonders. I am deeply grateful.

9. JENNIFER F.

My husband and I were blessed to easily conceive our first child the first month we tried. It was a healthy and easy pregnancy until 39 weeks. I checked into the hospital one week before my due date because I had several markers for preeclampsia at that point. I was induced very early the next morning; after the Pitocin drip started, the doctor observed signs of fetal distress whenever I contracted. She said that it was likely that the baby's cord was wrapped around his neck and I was prepped for a routine but emergency Caesarean. The procedure was remarkably quick. The cord had been wrapped around his neck, but there were no further complications and our healthy little boy was born with a perfect 10 Apgar score.

My Asherman's Syndrome journey began immediately after the delivery of our first child. As this was my first pregnancy, I didn't realize what followed was unusual. I knew that recovery would be slower from the Caesarean than if I had delivered vaginally. But I was given very little guidance from my doctor on what to look for or be concerned about after the operation. My milk came in quickly and breastfeeding was much more difficult than I had anticipated. I was quickly engorged and experiencing pain and a fever. The doctor's office said that this was normal and suggested applying hot and cold compresses. I experienced heavy bleeding with severe clots and was told that this would end in a few days. The bleeding did stop eventually and the breastfeeding became easier. Life with a newborn was exhausting; my immune system seemed to be suffering. I experienced illnesses I had never encountered before, including an ear infection and, later, an eye infection.

I nursed my son for seventeen months and my periods never resumed. At my annual exam, the nurse practitioner said that it was not unusual to not have a period when breastfeeding and that it could take up to six months after finishing breastfeeding for my period to resume. On my son's second birthday I went back to the doctor to see why I still was not getting a period. At this point, I was experiencing the tiniest bit of stringy, dark discharge about every 28 days. We had put a lot of effort into conceiving our first child. I spent months charting my basal temperatures and checking my cervical fluid to identify the ideal date for conception. Even now, with no periods, I could tell where I was in my monthly cycle from these same markers I had tracked before my pregnancy. My doctor dismissed that I could know anything about my ovulation from the texture of cervical fluids, and she suggested I try a drug called Clomid to regulate my cycle and force ovulation if I wanted to try to conceive again. It was shocking to me that a doctor (particularly a female doctor) would be so dismissive of a patient's instincts about their own body. While this was my first experience with fertility issues, I found it difficult to fathom that any doctor's first course of treatment would be to prescribe a round of drugs. Always the researcher, I declined her offer of Clomid, went home to the Internet and started asking friends for a recommendation for a new doctor.

I found a wonderful new doctor that spent considerable time reviewing my history and talked to me about the process that he recommended for evaluating what could be causing my amenorrhea, or lack of menstruation. First, he ordered a simple set of basic blood tests to assess my fertility. These included a day three FSH (follicle stimulating hormone) test to check the quantity and quality of my egg reserve, an LH (luteinizing hormone) test, which would measure the hormone that helps the body release eggs each cycle, and finally, a test to measure the prolactin levels in my blood (which the doctor suggested might still be high as a result of the breastfeeding). Later that month, we also tested my progesterone levels and confirmed that I had ovulated. It was a relief that these tests came back with good results, but we still didn't know why I wasn't menstruating.

The next step, according to my new doctor, was to check my husband's sperm quality. I had done some additional research online and found information about Asherman's Syndrome. My doctor said that Asherman's was an unlikely diagnosis given my history, but that it was possible, as I had delivered by Caesarean. Next, he ordered a hysterosalpingogram (HSG) test to x-ray my uterus and fallopian tubes, mostly to ease my mind and rule Asherman's Syndrome out definitively. Everyone was surprised when there was absolutely no fill of my uterine cavity. I left the hospital with no test results, but I couldn't shake the sinking feeling that "no results" actually meant something in this case. My doctor called later that afternoon to confirm the presence of scar tissue, a probable cause of the amenorrhea.

My doctor said that he had treated Asherman's Syndrome before, but that it wasn't something that he had seen often. He suggested referring me to another doctor to perform surgery to remove the scar tissue. I scheduled what would be my first hysteroscopy and laparoscopy with a reproductive endocrinologist. Based on my history, we were all hoping for the best case scenario: a mild form of Asherman's Syndrome with scar tissue blocking the entrance to my uterus that could quickly and easily be removed. What we found was that my uterus was almost completely sealed shut with dense scarring. I had the most severe form of Asherman's Syndrome. The reproductive endocrinologist could not even find the openings to either of my fallopian tubes and had never seen a case of Asherman's that severe. Her recommendation to me was to consider adoption or surrogacy.

Again, I turned to the Internet for research. I found information about a doctor who treated Asherman's Syndrome regularly. I compiled all of the results from my recent fertility tests, the films from my HSG and a surgery report and sent it to this "expert." He called me as soon as he had all of my files and said that he believed he could reopen the uterus and remove the scar tissue from in front of my tubes. He had seen similar cases before and, although rare, they were caused when the walls of the uterus were sutured together following a Caesarean. Over the two years since my son's birth, my uterus had completely grown shut from the suture. I scheduled a second surgery with this new doctor. He reopened my uterus six months after my first procedure (three and a half years after my C-section) and was able to remove the scar tissue from in front of one fallopian tube, which was now functional.

For a month and a half after the surgery I took high doses of estrogen followed by a few days of progesterone. I found an acupuncturist who specialized in fertility issues and saw her weekly for acupuncture. I found an herbalist who specialized in fertility and saw her bi-weekly for uterine massage and warm castor oil packs. I drank raspberry leaf tea every day and took a daily CoQ10 (Coenzyme Q10) because I read that it could help regenerate my lining by increasing the blood flow to the uterus. My Asherman's Syndrome diagnosis became a full-time job.

After finishing the progesterone pills, I waited for my first period since my pregnancy. Unfortunately, all I got was three days of extremely painful cramps. My uterus was now open and my lining was regenerating, but it was likely that some scarring had reoccurred and was trapping the lining that should have been shed with my monthly cycle. This was causing the painful cramps. While the regrowth of scar tissue after surgery is not uncommon, it was promising that we could verify with ultrasounds that the majority of my uterus remained open.

I rescheduled a third procedure with the same doctor who had made some progress with the last surgery. This hysteroscopy and laparoscopic surgery confirmed that a small band of scar tissue had grown back. The doctor removed the scarring again. This time, following a month and a half of hormones and another round of the alternative treatments, I finally had my first period in almost five years.

I had a follow-up HSG to confirm that my uterus looked good; this time the film showed my uterus filling with the dye that went up and through my one fallopian tube. My local obstetrician and my wonderful new Asherman's surgeon declared that my uterus was "good enough" to try and conceive. My husband and I were encouraged to begin trying as soon as possible in the event that there might be some re-scarring.

In spite of my age (39 years) and having only the one functioning fallopian tube, we conceived that first month.

My second pregnancy was as uneventful as the first. My obstetrician ordered several ultrasounds and we watched the pregnancy with great caution. As I had had three hysteroscopic surgeries in the year prior to my pregnancy, he monitored my cervix so that, if it appeared to weaken or open, a cerclage (cervical stitches) could be placed to help hold the cervix shut until delivery. Because of the Asherman's and my age, I also saw a perinatalogist. The perinatalogist scanned high-resolution ultrasounds for signs that the placenta had attached to scar tissue (accreta), which could mean a hysterectomy would be necessary at delivery. He also watched for bands of scar tissue that could break away and rupture the embryonic sac as my uterus slowly expanded. Thankfully, none of these issues materialized.

My obstetrician advised a final amniocentesis to ensure the baby's lungs were developed and then schedule a delivery for 37 weeks. I delivered a beautiful baby girl via another (this time scheduled) Caesarean. The placenta was easily and fully delivered afterwards with no signs of accreta and only a small amount of visible scar tissue where my original C-section scar appeared. Recovery from the second Caesarean was remarkably easier. It has been over a year since our daughter was born. I recently stopped nursing and am confident that I will return to a normal cycle again.

10. JENNIFER G.

My Asherman's journey began the day I went in for a routine D&C to remove a polyp. I was 32 years old at the time. I had no children and never had any pregnancies. I was in a two-year relationship. I always wanted children and finally found the man of my dreams that I wanted to have children with. I do remember my OB/GYN talking to me about the procedure and said there were very little risks with the surgery. Honestly, I do not even remember if Asherman's was even mentioned. I didn't really take any of those risks seriously. After all, my mom who had six pregnancies and multiple D&C's due to other issues never had any problems. My sister had four children and also had many D&Cs performed. I had nothing to worry about, right? That day I didn't realize that a simple procedure could drastically and permanently change my life both physically and mentally.

After my D&C, months went by and I had no period. Before the D&C, I always had a period every month like clockwork. I questioned my doctor and asked why I was not having one. He blamed it on my birth control. I had been on birth control for several years before and after the D&C. I didn't quite understand how that could affect it, except for my lining being a bit thinner on birth control. After all, my period was normal while I was on birth control before the D&C, and I knew the exact day I would start. I had not missed a period since I started when I was 13 years old. I believed him, because he was the doctor and I trusted him. Many months later still nothing. He did blood work to look at my hormone levels. Everything came back normal. Finally he decided to do a hysterosalpingogram (HSG). This procedure involves a catheter inserted into the cervix, dye is instilled up into the cervix and uterine cavity. It is used to visualize any scarring, polyps, adhesions, or blockages within your fallopian tubes or uterus. It also reveals the shape and size of your uterus and fallopian tubes. The test is used primarily to diagnose fertility problems; however, sometimes the procedure itself will loosen up any tissue or debris that may be causing an obstruction or blockage.

He made several attempts to do the procedure but could not. He told me it was because my uterus was tilted and there was nothing to be concerned about. I believed him and didn't think anymore of the actual procedure. Looking back now, that's when I started to prepare myself mentally that I would never have my own children. I knew deep down inside that something was just not right and it isn't normal for a woman my age to stop having a period?

Almost a year after my surgery I called to have my yearly exam done. The day I called was the day of my OB/GYN's funeral. My doctor was killed in an automobile accident. I was devastated. This doctor was young and had several children. My heart ached for his family. It was difficult to find a doctor like him. He was loved by all of his patients. The fact that he passed away affected me later on but for a different reason.

I still was not having a period and ended up going to the doctor that took my doctor's place after he passed. I talked to him about my concerns and he did more blood tests and told me not to worry. It was my birth control pills. I believed him and felt that we were not ready to have children yet and my career was going great at that time so no need to pursue. I heard from two doctors that it was because of my pill. Still, in the back of my mind though I felt that something wasn't right. I started telling people I would never have children and it just won't fit into my life. I did this to somewhat prepare myself for not being able to have children. I found out later you could never prepare for that, even though I started preparing for it early on.

One day my sister called me to let me know that her doctor told her about having an endometrial ablation to keep her from having periods. Her periods were very heavy and affected her life day to day. This was an option for her seeing she was finished having children. She asked me if I think that is what happened to me. That really got me thinking. I went off the birth control pill and I started looking for a new OB/GYN. One that I hoped would listen to me. I found one recommended by a co-worker of mine. I made an appointment with him and within 30 minutes of letting him know my history I was getting answers. He told me about this rare condition sometimes caused by an over aggressive D&C among other complications: Asherman's Syndrome. He told me not to worry and that one day he will deliver my baby. He sent me for another hysterosalpingogram to look at my uterus.

That day was the scariest day of my life. The technicians doing the procedure seemed to be having problems. They were whispering to each other and saying maybe we need to get a doctor. They kept apologizing as they were trying to force the catheter into my cervix. All I could think is what was wrong with me? Why can't they get in? She called another technician in to try. The pain was intense. They said they have never seen this before. Finally, they called a doctor in to try. After several failed attempts they told me they could not get into my cervix. I was in severe pain as well as scared. The looks of confusion on their faces didn't help either. They didn't know what to say or do for me. I tried to fight back the tears from the pain and the fear. Once I got into my car, I cried all the way home. I felt so alone and was wondering what could be wrong. Will they know what was wrong with me seeing they couldn't perform the tests?

I went back to my new doctor. He told me that I did indeed have Asherman's Syndrome and that my uterus is completely scarred shut. He set me up to go to a well-known fertility clinic. I later found out this fertility clinic really only specialized in IVF and not fixing problems that cause infertility. My visits to this RE were awful. My boyfriend never came to any appointments with me. I was also unaware at the time; I was at the mercy of a doctor that could not admit he did not know how to treat Asherman´s. He kept me on estrogen treatments for months to try to build up lining. He told me he was going to do a D&C to try to restore my uterus. I was even more confused. That is what caused my problem. Why would he do that procedure? The relationship between my boyfriend and me was quickly deteriorating. I went for weekly visits to check my lining and each week no change. Each week my boyfriend didn't ask me how it went. I would be upset and he just distanced himself from me. He changed the subject as if he didn't hear me.

My final visit with that reproductive endocrinologist was when he coldly told me I would never have children. He said I should have a hysterectomy. He said it as if it was not a big deal. I was so crushed. I couldn't stop crying. How could this be? Why is it so difficult? I thought I was prepared to hear this. I tried to convince myself that I didn't want kids. I told everyone I wanted a career instead. I did it to prepare for this very day. I found out that you couldn't prepare yourself for those words; no matter how it is told to you and what you think you believe, again I was so alone.

In the meantime, I went on the Web to look for information about Asherman´s Syndrome. There was not much information about AS. I did however find a group started by another woman that had her fertility stolen due to AS. There were many women like myself starving for information as well as many knowledgeable women that took control of their destiny by educating themselves and finding the right doctor to treat AS; Ashermans.org

I told them that my RE wanted to do a D&C and then a hysterectomy if that didn't work. He also told me I would NEVER have children of my own and I should consider surrogacy or adoption. I had several replies from the women telling me to find a doctor that can treat AS. This doctor did not know what he was doing. I was then recommended to a doctor from what was called an A LIST Doctor on the group. This is a doctor that successfully treated women with AS. At this time, I realized that doctors don't know everything. I no longer had trust in any doctor. I also realized that the doctor that caused my AS knew something was wrong and so did the doctor who took over his patients when he died. I was so angry with the doctor that died and the one that took his place as well as the first Reproductive Endocrinologist I met with. I felt guilt about being so angry with the doctor that caused my AS, but I was. He lied to me. They knew what was wrong and now I am 35 years old and probably will not ever have my own children! After getting my files from the practice, it clearly stated that he did not see a polyp but proceeded with the D&C anyway. That one decision has affected my life.

Meanwhile my relationship was really starting to struggle. I felt like my boyfriend didn't care. I was hurt so deeply inside. I was on the verge of tears all the time. My boyfriend didn't want to adopt and I knew we could not afford surrogacy or fertility treatments. I started dealing with my pain by shutting down. He never went with me to the doctor's I figured he would know that I needed him to go to the doctor with me. I was always the only woman in the waiting room sitting by herself without her partner by her side. I sat there with envy holding back tears hoping no one could see my pain. I was alone when I was told I wouldn't have children. I just couldn't prepare myself for those words. It is a hollow empty feeling, to know that you will never hear 'mommy' or 'I love you' from your child. I felt like my soul was ripped out when the doctor told me that.

I was just so angry at everything and everyone. I decided to confront the doctor that took my other doctor's place. I wanted so badly to talk to my doctor that passed. I even considered visiting his grave. I knew that his children lost their father and his wife lost her husband. Who am I to be angry with him? I knew he would be sad to know that he caused my AS and my infertility. I decided I needed to forgive him and that confronting the other doctor would help me get past my anger and hopefully help other women. My hope was he wouldn't ignore the signs as time is of the essence when it comes to women and their chances of having children. I lost 3 ½ years. They needed to know that estrogen treatments should be given before and after the D&C. I made an appointment to see the doctor as if it was a routine exam. I looked forward to this moment to get some closure. I had two letters one for him to read along as I read to him. My hands trembled so much and I broke down. I asked him to read it. He read it and denied my claims, but I expected that. I knew it bothered him. He was blindsided by this letter, the same way I was blindsided when I was told I wouldn't be able to have children. I asked him to listen to women when they tell him something isn't right along with the obvious signs. I felt so empowered after that meeting. My anger was gone!

I started going to my new RE who was recommended to me by another woman in the support group. He was the first one to ask me how I was doing. I sobbed and told him I was not doing well at all. He put me on estrogen again to try to build up lining. After months of estrogen and no lining improvement he did my first surgery in M arch of 2005 that opened up my uterus. I still did not have a period.

My relationship ended with my boyfriend. I started to see a counselor who deals in infertility recommended by my doctor. I went to her every two weeks for several months. I had one more surgery the following December to remove the rest of the scar tissue. It got to the point that I couldn't stand to see pregnant women and babies. While I was happy for them, I was hurt because I couldn't have my own. Even my best friend seemed to shy away and avoid the "fertility issue", never asking me about what was going on. I completely shut down and kept my pain inside. I had many nights that I just sobbed while posting my pain on the support group website. The ladies in the group were the only ones I could trust and that could understand what I was living with.

The counseling made me realize that my boyfriend didn't know how to help me. He felt I would be sad if we talked about it. Men are wired differently. When they can't fix it, they shy away from it. I also realized that the breakdown of our relationship was my own personal struggles. I didn't communicate and tell him that I needed him. He was hurt and confused when we broke up. We were always great communicators and best friends. We could talk for hours on end and laugh. He thought I left him for someone else. He didn't see that he hurt me by not supporting me. After counseling I realized I wanted our relationship back so bad.

Finally I got up enough nerve to tell him I missed him and that I wanted him back. We got back together after nine months of being apart. On April 29th, 2006 we spent our second weekend together and we knew that we were going to be together forever! It was like old times. We agreed to communicate what we needed. I vowed to never give up on us again. We grew and became a better and stronger couple because of this AS journey.

In August of 2006 we went to meet with my RE to discuss the probability of having children and risks involved. My doctor felt that the reward would outweigh the risks involved and talked about the possibility of needing assistance. It was the first time we went to the doctor together. We decided that we would try starting in December and said that we would try before looking at any possible obstacles. We also planned to get married.

On October 4th, 2006, I woke up with this feeling that I can't explain. I felt pregnant. I don't know how because I had never been pregnant before but something told me to take a pregnancy test. I took the test. It immediately showed that I was pregnant! I was shocked and must have looked at it 100 times. I was scared and excited! My fiancé didn't believe it when I told him. He wanted to be sure before he got his hopes up. He was cautiously optimistic.

We went for our first ultrasound the following Monday. We didn't see anything but a gestational sac and nothing else. My doctor said I would probably miscarry. He had me come back the following week for another ultrasound. I was so devastated and cried for two days. I could not face anyone at work as they did not know what was happening and I knew if someone asked what is was wrong I would just crumble and break down. I kept my office door closed and consumed myself with work. I prayed a lot and found the hope I needed to stay strong. After all, I felt very pregnant and I knew this was going to be a viable pregnancy. My fiancé was very concerned about my hope. He felt I was setting myself up for a big fall.

That day finally came. It was finally our turn. We watched the monitor and saw a heartbeat!!!!!!!!! 100 BEATS PER MINUTE!!! My doctor felt it still might not be a viable pregnancy. I went back every week until I made it to week 12 of my pregnancy. My doctor monitored me closely throughout my pregnancy, which helped me stay hopeful. I had a wonderful pregnancy. My fiancé and I went to classes about breast-feeding and C-sections together. We were doing things that we would have never done before AS. I believe that all of the heartache we had was so that we could share this wonderful miracle together. I would tell him when I wanted him to come to the doctor with me and he knew I needed him there. In fact he wanted to be there. My faith, the renewed relationship and this miracle we were experiencing gave me so much strength and hope. We were closer than we had ever been. We planned to marry on April 29th.

Week 32 I was having contractions. I thought they were Braxton Hicks but they seemed to be more frequent and regular. On April 23rd I was at 33 weeks, I left work to go to the doctor and he told me to get to the hospital that I was 2cm dilated and 100% effaced. I spent the next week in the hospital getting steroid shots and medication to keep me from having her too early. Through the week I wrote in my journal that I kept since I found out I was pregnant. It didn't matter to me that I was laid up in bed. I just wanted to keep my baby safe and give her the best possible chance when entering this world. The doctor told me we had to get to at least 34 weeks and she would have a great chance with limited time in the NICU. I was hopeful at times and scared at other times when the contractions would start back up. The baby never showed any sign of stress through the entire time I was having contractions. She stayed strong and so did I. I knew in time I would hold my daughter.

At 34 weeks, on April 29th, the labor could not be stopped and they set me up for a C-section. My doctor who had diagnosed me with AS and had told me that he would deliver my baby one day came in on his day off to deliver my daughter with the doctor on call. He promised me he would and he did. My beautiful miracle was born weighing 6lb 3oz. Isabella was in the NICU mainly for formality due to her gestational age of 34 weeks and also her glucose levels. After 24 long hours I finally got to hold the baby I had always dreamed of having. I could not believe I became a mother. She is perfect. We brought our healthy beautiful bundle of joy home three days after she was born. We ended up getting married on her due date of June 10th seeing she was born on the day we planned to marry. Those sleepless nights were the greatest nights of my life. Her presence in our life is truly the most amazing blessing we have ever had. She is now 2 ½ and I still cannot believe I am her mother.

I breastfed for a year. I still have not had a period, but have been experiencing something very different than I was prior to my pregnancy. I went for a hydro-sonogram and was diagnosed with adenomyosis. This is a condition that causes severe pain throughout the month. A pregnancy, if one can be obtained, would be extremely risky. I was told that hysterectomy is the only cure. So now I am at the end of my road. I am hoping to find a doctor that can remove the adenomyosis to avoid hysterectomy. I still would not be able to ever have children, but I will not have the problems that go along with hysterectomy. My heart is aching to have one more. I am experiencing the same feelings of anger, sadness and isolation I went through when I was first diagnosed with Asherman´s. I was given hope with one miracle. I guess I had hoped for one more. I couldn't understand why someone would not be satisfied with one child. After all at least they had one. Now I understand. It hurts more now, because I know how truly wonderful it is to have a child and to experience such a wonderful miracle. Something I will never experience again. I know that it doesn't end here with my physical pain and emotional pain. The physical pain will hopefully be gone soon, but the mental pain never will. How can one D&C cause so much heartache and pain?

11. SUE

The two most important things to remember when you are faced with fertility issues are to trust your own instincts, and, if you don't feel that your medical advisors are up to scratch, either get a second opinion or (preferably) get advice from the best experts you can find.

My Asherman´s journey began when I was newly married, aged 35 and desperate to get on with starting a family. We had an easy start with me falling pregnant within two months of the wedding, much to the joy of my husband and I. Unfortunately at our 3 month scan we received the terrible news that I had suffered what is termed a 'missed miscarriage'- a 'blighted ovum' in medical speak which essentially meant that the baby had died but the pregnancy sac had kept growing and my body had not expelled the 'products of conception' in the normal manner of a miscarriage.

Obviously the news was a terrible shock, and I was keen to try and recover from the miscarriage as quickly and easily as possible. I was given some choices at this point that I wish I had been better informed about. For instance I didn't know that the hormonal levels of someone who is 3 months pregnant are much higher than someone who has a D&C (dilation and curettage to remove the products of conception) at 4 or 6 weeks. This then puts you at a higher risk – because your body takes longer to produce the hormones that will start a period – of scarring in the uterus. I took the doctor´s advice that there was 'virtually no risk' in having a D&C and opted for this operation because I felt I could not face taking an abortion pill and effectively giving birth to my unformed baby, or simply waiting – however long it took – for my body to expel the pregnancy sac of its own accord. However knowing what I do now, both of those options would have been infinitely preferably to the nightmare journey that the D&C option took me on.

I have since learned that a D&C should always be avoided, unless there is no alternative. Certainly in the area I was treated it is policy for D&C's to be performed on an 'emergency' list, so someone newly qualified, and certainly not a specialist is liable to perform the operation. It is also not policy to issue estrogen which is one way to prevent scarring occurring should the womb have been damaged in what is actually a relatively risky procedure.

What followed was 18 months of trying to convince my medical carers that the D&C had caused some sort of damage. Despite having fallen pregnant so easily the first time I was having no luck post operation. There is obviously procedure to follow, hormonal tests and hoops of that nature to jump through. Through a contact at the local hospital I came under specialist care much more quickly than is usual. Although this did little to speed the diagnosis of Asherman´s, in fact my specialist was so resistant to the idea that the D&C had caused any damage that coming under his care may well have been more of a hindrance than a help.

Due to lower abdominal pain and remarkably light periods I was concerned fairly early on that there was an issue following the D&C. Alongside hormonal tests I was sent for other diagnostic tests that were unrelated to fertility, including a colonoscopy for Irritable Bowel Syndrome. In this manner the first six months following the miscarriage were eaten up.

I then embarked on monthly ultrasounds that showed my endometrial lining thickening before my period in an uneven manner, and not thickening sufficiently to support a pregnancy. Clomid was issued to encourage the production of eggs and to encourage the lining to thicken, and this was issued in ever increasing amounts, until I was attending a fertility clinic (at great expense) and injecting huge amounts of drugs that I did not need. It seemed to be flying in the face of common sense as far as I could see, because I had fallen pregnant so easily the first time. So all the while I questioned the role the D&C had played in my fertility issues and was told at every turn that complications following a D&C were 'highly unlikely'.

Mentally I really struggled, I attended counselling and faced up to the possibility that I may not be able to conceive children naturally. It really was the darkest period of my life. Had I not had such a supportive husband and also amazing support from my friends and family it would have been almost impossible to bear.

I finally sought a second opinion. I discussed my concern around the D&C, the patchy quality of my periods that had followed the operation and the lack of endometrial lining on the ultrasound. Within the space of a 10 minute conversation I was advised that it was almost certainly the D&C that had caused my fertility issues and that the easiest course of action to determine this was to have an HSG – a hysterosalpingogram - which effectively x-rays the womb and tube entrances to check for 'adhesions' (scarring). On the strength of this conversation I discovered I had Asherman's and was able to tap into the support group and locate expert advice and opinions.

By this time my specialist at the local hospital had run out of viable options and scheduled me in for a hysteroscopy, which operates to look at the womb, with the option to remove any adhesions by scope. Newly armed with my Asherman's support I discovered that a local NHS specialist had worked with one of the 'A list' Asherman's experts and therefore I felt comfortable with being put on his surgical list. To cut a long story short the surgery found extensive adhesions which was able to be removed by scope, their removal was confirmed by a second HSG. Following surgery I was put on 2 months estrogen therapy to prevent re-scarring and was then given the green light to try and conceive. Which I did, the first month we tried.

A post Asherman´s pregnancy can have complications and I spent a nervous first few months with periodic brown spotting. I also suffered with a severe irritable uterus which I personally suspect may have something to do with my history, but I have yet to establish this as a certainty. This caused preterm labor whereby my son was born just over 7 weeks early. Post Asherman´s pregnancies are also at risk of the placenta adhering to the womb, which mine did in part following the birth of my son. This required a further D&C under my Asherman´s trained specialist and required more estrogen treatment which made breastfeeding problematic but not impossible with the help of a drug called Domperidnone, which successfully counteracted the effects of the estrogen on my milk supply.

My son, Eli, is now 15 months old and is living proof that there is life after Asherman´s. He is beautiful, and I thank God every day that I was lucky enough to conceive him. I am doubly blessed as I write this from the confinement of the couch where I am pregnant with my second child, the irritable uterus and extended confinement a small price to pay for the joy that is motherhood.

As I said at the beginning … my advice to anyone who is struggling with fertility issues is to trust your instincts and don't rest until you can also trust your doctor.

12. JENNIFER H.

A MIRACLE OF THE TINIEST PROPORTIONS

The doctor who told me to have a hysterectomy peered at me from over the edge of my medical file. It was December and his office was unusually cold. Two weeks earlier, I had had a hysterosalpingogram (HSG), a radiological exam where fluoroscopic dye is injected into the uterus to check for blocked tubes and other reproductive abnormalities. On some occasions it will also detect other blockages in the uterus. In my case, the dye could not pass beyond my cervix because scar tissue had occluded my womb from the top by my fallopian tubes down to my cervix.

The medical resident performing the exam had tried to inflate a balloon in my uterus, just past the top of my cervix, as is standard procedure. This tiny balloon usually creates a seal so that dye can flow freely up to a woman's fallopian tubes, showing a nice, normal uterine structure. In my case, the balloon inflated in my cervix, forcibly dilating it and feeling much like early labor. This happened because the adhesions in my uterus were so thick that nothing could get through, not even a tiny balloon on the end of a probe.

At the time, I recall thinking that the resident was doing something wrong and must not have had enough experience to perform the exam. After all, I was at a top teaching hospital where well-respected doctors oversaw all procedures. The nurse that day even took great pains to explain to me that what had happened was likely a minor complication in procedure, and that I should ask for a second exam with the physician in charge or a reproductive specialist. I left the exam mildly concerned but completely ignorant to the severity of my condition.

At my follow-up appointment, I learned that I had Asherman's Syndrome. The doctor told me, "In some cases we can cut the adhesions, but in your condition there is no way to know where the planes of the uterus are. If we begin cutting, we might perforate your uterus or cut the veins within the tissue." He went on to explain that cases like mine usually require a hysterectomy because of the potential for endometriosis, where the uterine lining begins to grow *outside* the uterus, causing pain and sometimes serious internal bleeding.

It seemed I sat there for ten minutes without saying a word.

My husband and I did not want it to end in that room, with that doctor. We wanted another child, and I did not believe that our dreams could end without any discussion. I began looking for more information because with information comes options. I was determined to find a way out of the Asherman's corner.

I had had no trouble conceiving my son. There was nothing extraordinary about my pregnancy or delivery. But I had to have a D&C two months postpartum due to retained placenta. I found out later that this was the delicate healing time for the uterus. Having a D&C so soon after delivery could cause the uterus to grow scar tissue, not healthy endometrial tissue.

Shortly after my condition was confirmed, I found a support group on the Internet of women who had Asherman's Syndrome (www.ashermans.org). Some of those women had undergone successful operations to remove the scar tissue and had eventually had children. Many women, like me, reeled after learning their diagnosis. We aired our sorrows in a Yahoo group and shared stories, grief, and nuggets of valuable information and encouragement that we hoped would help us get pregnant.

On Poly Spyrou's Ashermans.org website, I found two "A-list" specialists in California. As soon as I could, I scheduled an appointment to meet one of them, who was only a few hours away from our home—a lucky turn that would prove helpful in future months.

When the official diagnosis and report from the hospital made its way to my obstetrician, she told me that my chances of overcoming Asherman's and my chances of conceiving were nil. She told me I was too old and there was no chance that my uterus would recover enough to grow a lining, even if the scar tissue could be safely removed. She was doomsayer number two. The voice in my head told me that she was ill informed.

In my typically optimistic manner, which was growing more resolute each day, I stopped seeing her and found a new, more positive obstetrician. He encouraged me to meet with the specialist who said he could repair my uterus. *This* was the kind of person I needed on my team. He believed in miracles.

Perhaps I was naive or woefully ignorant to the severity of my situation, but that is the thing about hope. One has to be blind to pessimism or it will drag you down. I elected to find people who would share my optimism (or at least indulge my naiveté), because they would look for solutions and not automatically tell me to go home and cry. Rather than dwell on the delay in diagnosis and the poor treatment I received from the university fertility clinic that had performed the HSG, I decided to focus on success. I poured my energy into my condition and began to look for a solution. I needed to clear the scar tissue from my uterus and my mind. I needed positive influences and information. I needed a doctor who could correct my condition.

The A-list specialist who was three hours from my home had hundreds of successful hysteroscopic surgeries to his credit. He was a prolific writer and speaker on the subject and had an anything-is-possible attitude. I liked him from the first moment we met. We spent a few minutes explaining our history, and then he pulled out my HSG images. After a cursory glance, he dismissed them. "Films mean nothing," he told me. "I need to see this for myself, so let's just get to it." After he confirmed my condition with an ultrasound exam, we discussed treatment, and then scheduled my first surgery for two weeks from then.

This specialist did five hysteroscopic surgeries under conscious sedation, followed by high doses of estrogen to encourage endometrial growth. A week after each surgery, the doctor checked my uterus to see if the area was still open. After a few weeks of healing, he performed another surgery. My sixth and final surgery was completed at a local fertility clinic, where I had access to reproductive assistance with fertility drugs and artificial insemination.

Healing is not only physical, however. I believe that the mind and spirit play equal parts in helping a body recover. Early in the process of my surgeries, I started going through hypnotherapy training with a woman who specializes in working with infertile couples. Not only did this amazing lady teach me relaxation and visualization techniques, she was a valuable resource for navigating the medical system and the various diagnostic tests, surgeries, and fertility services I would need.

Throughout this yearlong struggle, I had moments of deep despair and disappointment, but underneath all the sadness was an overwhelming feeling that another child was waiting to join our family. I could not shake the little voice in my head, and the more I heard it, the stronger my conviction grew. I credit the ability to tune into this voice to my hypnotherapist, who helped buoy my spirits and taught me to focus on a successful conception and birth. Under her guidance, I practiced visualizing a healthy baby girl. She was so alive to me that I would dream about her blonde hair and could see her taking little, shaky toddler steps. In my mind's eye, I could see her struggling in her car seat or watching *Handy Manny* on television while playing in our family room. She was destined to be on this earth, and no amount of pessimism or gloomy prognoses could deter me.

Ultimately, I conceived twins, with the help of artificial insemination and fertility drugs. The drugs pushed my ovaries to produce three follicles that were large enough to release eggs. Two of those eggs fertilized and then settled themselves into my very thin endometrium for what was supposed to be a joyous pregnancy. I did not, however, carry both of my babies to term.

One of our babies, Julianne, was lost at nineteen weeks of gestation. To save our remaining baby, Beth, I was hospitalized and confined to my bed for seven weeks, while we fought early labor and the risk of infection. The journey was not easy. The medications were hard on my body and the emotional pain my husband, young son, and I endured threatened to suffocate us. Beth, however, held on until twenty-six weeks and was born weighing just under two pounds.

The story of saving Beth is nothing short of miraculous—but we are familiar with miracles. It was a miracle that I conceived. It was a miracle that one of our babies was saved. Beth is now four years old, perfect in every detail, vibrant, healthy, and full of the same piss and vinegar that helped me fight Asherman's Syndrome.

13. PAIGE

August 7, 2006: By all accounts, a very joyous day. A very liberating day. A very proud day. A day that I would rejoice and marvel at the wonders on this earth. A day that took three and a half long, painstaking years to arrive. A day that I owe so much to so many before me. A day that I forgave. A day of rejoicing. A day of new beginnings. A day that will forever be etched in my mind as one of the best days of my life. You see, he wasn't supposed to be here. By the true sense of the word, he is my little miracle. What had transpired from a routine dilation and curettage (D&C) eight years prior became a long, treacherous, emotional journey. One we almost didn't make. After the birth of my daughter in 2002 – a routine delivery but with placenta delivery complications – I required two D&Cs: one at the time of delivery, and another emergency surgery five days later. One could possibly say that I am not even supposed to be here. But, for some strange reason, I made it through and healed quite nicely. Or so we thought. Only minimal periods after nine months of breastfeeding and taking the mini-pill, but my doctor was not concerned; he chalked it up to breastfeeding. At my yearly checkup, we discussed the possibilities of carrying another child. The doctor didn't see why not, there was no evidence of placenta accreta in the pathology reports. Conceiving and carrying a baby to term were not the issue – delivery was. So, I went home and shared the great news with my husband and we began trying immediately. After six months, nothing had happened. This time the doctor said since I had hit the 35-year marker, it may take longer and to give it six more months. Again, nothing, except my periods had officially diminished and were very painful.

January 14, 2004: By all accounts, a horrific day. A very depressing day. A very humbling day – I was damaged merchandise. A day that I would grow to resent. A day that I grew resentful. A day that took away all my hopes and dreams. A day that I crumbled and was crippled. A day that saw more tears than I had ever dreamed possible. A day that will forever change me in more ways than I knew possible. You see, it wasn't supposed to be here. By the sounds of the words, it was my cancer – Asherman's Syndrome (AS). During a sonohysterogram (SHG), the doctor could not get the instrument past my cervix. The pain was horrific. After several attempts, I was told to get dressed and meet the doctor in his office. As I entered, I found him fumbling in his medical book and then searching his computer. After a few minutes, and with a very sorrowful look on his face, he proceeded to tell me I had AS. I thought, 'okay, what is that? It's treatable, right?' He then handed me two brochures – one on hysteroscopies, the other on hysterectomies and explained that they could try and fix the scarring, but mine seemed very severe, he was not optimistic. It was a short conversation in the big scheme of things. One that still haunts me. I got sent home with the two pamphlets, not really knowing what I had been diagnosed with or how I got it. 'Is it like cancer? Did my body do this? Why? Why?' I spent the next few months researching all I could get my hands on about AS. I was very shocked to learn that someone did this to me, even though it was unknowingly and not maliciously. After all, I was here. I made it through a difficult delivery and have two beautiful children who need me.

Through my research, I discovered an online International Support Group (www.ashermans.org), which armed me with all the necessary information I needed to know to move forward in tackling this devastating news. Over the course of the next two years, I had surgeries performed by Dr. David Lee at OHSU and Dr. Charles March at California Fertility

Partners in Los Angeles, along with numerous recannalization surgeries performed by Dr. Amy Thurmond at Epic Imaging in Portland, OR. I was told I had the worst case seen (99.9% scarred shut past the cervix). Treatment included high dosages of Premarin and Estrace to build up the lining of my uterus along with balloon stents to keep the uterus open. We spent close to $7,000 out-of-pocket to have me functioning as a woman again and when one tube wouldn't remain open, I was advised to use in vitro fertilization (IVF) – not an option for us both ethically and financially.

In 2005, my family moved to Dallas, Texas where Dr. James Madden, RE and Infertility Medical Director at Dallas Presbyterian Healthcare System, proved that my ovary on my good tube side was functioning, that my uterus looked "brand new", and gave us the positive reinforcement and encouragement that we could conceive naturally. I guess I only needed to hear some positive news for a change. Two months later, we were pregnant – one month before we were going to give up all hope and call it good. Just as I was beginning to accept that my family was complete the way it was.

Even though this road I have traveled has been most difficult, I no longer have ill feelings towards what transpired, believe me this was a long healing process. This would be true even if I didn't have my little miracle. I do not wish what I went through for any other woman. However, I have learned so much – about myself, the world of medicine, and the power of positive thinking and healing – that has helped me to be a better person, wife and mother. It has made me stronger and for that, in a strange way, I thank Drs. Thomas O. Flath and Charles Neilson who basically saved my life so I could be here for my children.

Preston Elliot Jezek was born August 7, 2006. My little miracle post AS baby. He completes me.

14. PAULA

After my son was born in 2004, I heard one question repeated by strangers and friends: "How was your labor?"

To some, I'd smile serenely and say, "Oh, fine. Long, but fine." My friends would get the gory details of my 36-hour-labor and 45-minutes of pushing that ended with the obstetrician pulling out the remnants of my placenta in pieces. The surreal buzz I felt holding my newborn was interrupted by the realization that the obstetrician was looking at my afterbirth on a tray, trying to determine if I had passed all the tissue. I remember suddenly feeling dizzy and saying repeatedly, "I can't breathe, why can't I breathe?" The attending nurse shushed me and held an oxygen mask on my face, telling me to take deeper breaths. It was soon over, and my fatigue took charge.

Looking back, I should have paid attention to the first red flag: retained placenta. Many Asherman's cases start with exactly what had happened in my Labor & Delivery room. But I only recall my blissful love for the new little person I had helped usher into the world; my son's eyes were the only thing I focused on.

Two-weeks into my 'new mommy'-ness, I was still bleeding; on the day of my first post-natal checkup, I was dining with my husband and our new little bundle. When lunch ended, I stood up, and suddenly froze.

"What's wrong?" my husband asked.

"Take me home. I have to cancel my appointment." I called the doctor's office in a panic to reschedule for the next day. "I'm supposed to come to the office right now, but I just bled through my pants. Can I come tomorrow?" The nurse put me on hold.

"Paula?" It was the doctor. "If you're bleeding heavily, I want to see you right away. Don't go home."

At the office, I undressed and waited for the exam to be over, all the while wondering if I should nurse my son before or after I left the office.

"You need an ultrasound." The doctor couldn't determine the source of my bleeding. With her limited office scan and with a broken placenta, she thought I was possibly retaining tissue that was causing hemorrhaging. She quickly wrote a referral and sent me to the imaging office, which was two short blocks away.

As a new mom, my only focus was my child. I was inexperienced in the 'things that can go wrong' in labor, and there was no chapter in my "What to Expect" book that talked about retained placenta. So I was blissfully ignorant of what I might be facing when I dutifully headed down the street to the ultrasound office, my son and husband in tow.

After my examination, the technician conferred with the doctor, and the decision was made to send me for a D&C that evening. "Why?" I asked. I was told that the D&C was *routine* for retained placenta, and that like most out-patient procedures, mine would take only a few hours of my time. I walked across the street to the hospital and filled out my admitting forms. I was given a surgery time of 7 pm. My husband was facing a few hours alone with our son, and hospital waiting rooms are no place to be alone, so I called my friend Lauren to keep him company and help hold the baby. She arrived just in time to see me walk out of the surgical prep area in my flimsy gown.

"Ok guys, have fun!" I said cheerfully as I walked past the double doors further into the hospital surgery suite.

The next thing I recall is crying on the recovery table, with the doctor hovering over me. I asked how long I had been out, and learned that my surgery lasted over 7 hours. I was miserably cold, and confused as to why I felt so weak. A 'routine procedure' that was supposed to take three hours total from anesthesia to recovery lasted much longer. At one point, the doctors came to my husband and asked if he would give permission for a hysterectomy. He balked. The decision was made to simply place sterile cotton swabbing into my uterus—called 'packing'—to hopefully stop the blood flow. My uterus stopped bleeding eventually, and by 3 am I was stable enough to spend the night in surgical recovery, with two wonderfully compassionate nurses watching over me.

When I came to in the morning, I learned the full extent of what had happened. In the course of my procedure, I suddenly started to hemorrhage heavily. I lost a total of six units of blood (an average body of my size holds about four units at any given time) and required four units of transfusions. It was a full week before I felt strong enough to walk down the block without feeling lightheaded.

I've mentioned how ignorant I was of the many warning signs that something was wrong with my body. During the two weeks post birth and prior to my D&C, I was extremely weak. My happiness buoyed me past any exhaustion I felt; anything remotely negative I experienced was chalked up to my having had a marathon labor. The bleeding I experienced seemed normal; after all, the books I'd read mentioned that bleeding could last up to a month or so.

Then, the decision to have the D&C to treat retained placenta seemed perfectly acceptable to me, because all I heard were the words *"routine," "in a few hours and you'll be done."* Again, it was my first birth; everything I saw, said, heard, or felt was done so through the rose-colored love I had for my baby.

But as they say, hindsight is 20/20, and performing a D&C on a uterus that has recently experienced birth is almost always a precursor for developing Asherman's. Also, no one had thought to confer with me the fact that my broken placenta might have been caused by an accreta, when the placenta attaches too deeply into the uterine walls. Scraping the uterus with an accreta was sure to lead to traumatic bleeding.

On top of that, one of the major causal factors of Asherman's is a dilation and curettage; if the procedure is administered during the few weeks after giving birth, when the uterus is boggy and soft, the metal instruments will surely damage the uterine walls, which will lead to scarring—and an Asherman's diagnosis.

Which brings me to one year later, when I still had not resumed a menses. The obstetrician credited my lack of a period to breastfeeding. After a few more months, I successfully weaned my son, yet no period. The practice referred me to the network endocrinologist. I remember sitting across from him, still not fully recognizing what I was in store for. I explained I was sent for a consult due to my lack of a period, and he asked me for a history of my birth experience. I talked about the retained placenta, the bleeding, and the dilation and curettage.

Then it was his turn. He spoke in a low, steady voice, with very little emotion. I can't recall exactly what he said, because after he explained I likely had scarring which was occluding the opening of my cervix, he also said something about *"may not be able to have any more children."* That's all I heard that day.

I went through three subsequent surgeries in the five months following that initial meeting. The scarring was extensive, and my uterus was perforated during the first surgery. But, the scarring was removed for the most part, and I was able to conceive again with the help of IVF.

Today, my second son is just over a year old. I am still nursing, and have not had a period since he was born. I know I will be facing a few surgeries to correct Asherman's again, because my second birth experience was much like my first with broken placenta and extensive bleeding directly following the birth, except this time the decision was made to treat me with a uterine embolism.

What is more, this time, I am ready for what I'm now facing. I'm not ignorant of the complications, and I am confident in my ability to participate in the decisions that will be made on by behalf. **No woman should ever be blindsided by Asherman´s**—which is exactly what happens today when birth doesn't go exactly as they explain in 'the books,' and leads to a dilation and curettage.

There is a lack of dialog about Asherman's today, and a lack of knowledge about the dangers of electing a dilation and curettage, particularly soon after giving birth. This will almost always lead to scarring and complications related to infertility.

Right now Asherman's is thought to be under diagnosed. It is not documented as always leading to scarring although many of us are sure it does for a large proportion of women, although we cannot prove it.

Finding the Asherman's Yahoo! Group that Poly has started gave me resources to be able to ask questions and be ready for what I was facing after my initial consult with the endocrinologist.

Because birth is almost never 'by the book,' uterine scarring and Asherman's must become part of the dialog surrounding birth and birthing complications—it's the responsibility of us as a group to help make this happen.

15. MANDY

I had a baby girl in December 2004. My placenta broke at delivery and my original OB/GYN tried to manually remove it. However he did not get it all out, unknown to us. When I left the hospital, he gave me no warning signs to look for, although I mentioned concern over my abdomen being swollen quite a bit more on one side. When I was three weeks postpartum I had to attend the Emergency Room due to excessive bleeding. Once they determined it was a retained placenta, my original OB/GYN was called in to give me an emergency D&C. I lost excessive amounts of blood (borderline transfusion) and was in recovery for hours as they pounded on my abdomen trying to get all the blood out. During this time I slipped in and out of consciousness because my blood pressure was so low, often reading 40/20 as the monitors would go off. My original OB/GYN mentioned post surgery that there was more retained products than he was expecting. A few days after the D&C I spiked fever and ended up with a uterine infection. After a one-week-stay in the hospital, I was sent home and told this, "should not", affect my future fertility.

I pumped to give my daughter breast milk until the middle of March, (four months old) after the hospitalization stay she would no longer take to the breast and I was challenged to make enough milk, likely a result of the retained placenta. Until March, I never even worried about not starting my period because of the breastfeeding. In March I started on the birth control pill and after two rounds, still no period. I went back to my original OB/GYN specialist who was not concerned.

I still felt something was not right so I sought a second opinion. OB/GYN #2 immediately mentioned Asherman's Syndrome and recommended a hysteroscopy to see what was going on. He tried to perform a hysteroscopy in June, 2005, however, there was so much scar tissue at the opening he was unable to get the instrument in there to even look around. He said he would feel more comfortable having a Reproductive Endocrinologist (RE) look at it and/or perform the surgery.

At this point I consulted with the Yahoo Asherman's group and Dr. March, an A lister, who we'd have to fly to (loved him, but was financially out of reach for us) and my original local RE, who actually helped us get pregnant with my darling daughter (only child at this point) with one round of Clomid. She seemed to know what she was talking about and speculated that I might just have scarring at the opening of the uterus/cervix. She used a vaginal ultrasound to conclude this which I now know is not an effective means of determining scar tissue. She put me on estrogen prior to surgery to help build up my lining. Another reason I went with her and believed her was that I had a dermoid cyst on my left ovary that she said could be the reason for my lack of periods. I looked it up online and dermoids can change your hormone levels and cause you to not have a period. I needed to have the cyst removed and with her the surgery would be covered on my insurance. I trusted her and chose to allow her, my original RE, to do a laparoscopy and hsysteroscopy on me in October 2006. She did successfully remove the cyst from my left ovary. She attempted to only remove the scar tissue from my cervix as my uterus looked so bad. She kept repeating the words "bad" and telling me how I needed to consider surrogacy and move on with my life. I was absolutely devastated, but I didn't want to put too much weight into what she said at this point because this was the same woman who told me she didn't even think I had Asherman's and my chances at future pregnancies were good. She also admitted that she had only treated one case such as mine and they ended up doing surrogacy. I did get a light period after this surgery twice. Once with hormone induction and once 26 days later in the middle of estrogen treatment. I thought this was a good sign.

I then contacted Dr. March, and of course loved him again and knew he was the one for me. Due to financial reasons, we set my surgery for the first of the year. I remained on the estrogen in order to continue to build up any lining I might still have, hence I had been on estrogen a very long time … off and on for about a year!!! Dr. March performed a successful surgery in which he removed 99% of my scar tissue that was covering 80% of my uterus - severe. He also found a very large bald spot, 60% of no endometrium below the scarring and said only time will tell if this would grow back. Both of my tubes were blocked with scar tissue and he was able to remove the scarring and open up the tubes. He also advised us that I might need another surgery, but it would just depend on how my body heals. If it didn't heal well and there was little improvement, he likely would not recommend further surgery. If there was improvement, it might be worth it to attempt again.

Due to a stomach virus, the splint only stayed in ten days (was recommended for 14) and two months of estrogen. I did bleed for about 5 weeks post surgery. Dr. March just told me that hormones, surgery, etc. can do crazy things to your body. We were concerned that the bleeding was the scars oozing out. After the hormone withdrawal, I had two days of brown spotting followed by eight days of a bright red, medium flow period. Again, I thought this was a good sign. I had not seen this much blood since prior to getting pregnant when I had "normal" periods. I went for my HSG (hysterosalpingogram) in which they could not get the cavity to fill, even though it went into my left tube. They said it was because of all the damage from surgeries, etc. The radiologist walked into the room and immediately said, Asherman's Syndrome. Dr. March said not to panic quite yet. The HSG was inconclusive and I was told by my new local RE (local RE #2) who was a top RE in the Houston area that it was because my uterus was so abnormal. He then started to contradict himself and tried to convince me to have surgery with him instead of Dr. March. I felt his ego was getting in the way of me letting a true expert take care of me. I did not feel comfortable and phoned Dr. March. I told Dr. March how I felt I was being misled and he found me a new place to have my HSG where a successful HSG was performed. Thirteen images were taken, both my tubes were open and about 35-40% of scarring remaining. Dr. March advised me that there was a 50/50 chance another surgery would get me to the point where it would be safe to try to conceive. I took a leap of faith and flew out to CA in May '06 for a second surgery with Dr. March. I also found a new local RE (local RE #3,) that had been trained by Dr. March and would not try to contradict him. After the hormone treatment, I was told that about 10% of scarring remained. One of my tubes appeared to be blocked, but Dr. March said it must have been a spasm because they were open after the first surgery, at the first HSG, and at the second surgery (he was right). I was then given the green light to try to conceive.

We tried naturally for three to four months. I was going in for mid-cycle scans with my local RE (#3). My lining would measure anywhere between 4 and 7 mm. I did not ovulate the first cycle (side effect of being on estrogen for so long) and then after I did, but did not get pregnant. Upon Dr. March's advice, we tried a round of Clomid with estrogen to counter balance the anti-estrogen effects. On my first cycle of Clomid in Nov/Dec 06, my lining measured 8 mm and I had a mature follicle on my right side (the one they tried to tell me was blocked, but Dr. March knew it was just a spasm from the dye.) I was given a shot of Ovidrel at my local RE's office and sent home for relations. On December 19, 2006 I found out I was pregnant. I endured red/brown spotting during weeks 5-9 due to a subchorionic hematoma. I also had a band of scar tissue inside the gestational sac that appeared at 8 weeks and was gone by 12. At 8 weeks my cervix was measuring short and at 10.5 weeks I had a cerclage (a stitch) placed in. Between 12 and 24 weeks my pregnancy was uneventful and my high risk OB/GYN thought we had a great outlook. At 24.5 weeks on Mother's Day 2007, my water broke. I was so scared! I honestly thought I would deliver that day and we'd lose my precious baby boy. I was put on complete bed rest in the hospital and told there was a 50% chance I'd deliver in the next 48 hours. They watched for contractions, signs of infection, fetal distress, and bleeding. We were able to hold out for 22 days and at one day shy of 28 weeks pregnant, I started showing signs of a uterine infection and my baby had to be delivered that day, June 4, 2007. I opted for a vaginal delivery since I had been told at EVERY ultrasound that the placenta did not look adhered to the uterine wall. I labored for 9 hours and after 3 pushes my precious baby boy entered this world weighing a whopping 3 pounds, 1.2 ounces, and 15 inches long … all large for his gestational age as he should have been around 2 pounds! After the delivery my high risk OB/GYN had to "dig" for my placenta to get it to come out, several times. I started gushing blood. It was adhered. I could feel the blood pouring out of me. He administered two rounds of drugs to stop the bleeding and it would not stop. It quickly turned to an emergency hysterectomy. My poor husband was scared to death!! I was awake during the whole procedure which, thankfully, went off without a hitch. I was in the hospital for a week following delivery due to a massive blood loss … (levels as low as the 4s) and recovery from the hysterectomy. My team of high risk OB/GYNs decided not to transfuse because there are some very rare complications with transfusions and they concluded that rare things happen to me. So, I was slowly building my levels back up—taking medicine, vitamins, and eating red meat constantly. I was not too sad about the uterus being gone as I was done having children, but the recovery, etc., was not pleasant. My precious baby boy was in the level III NICU where he stayed until August 16, 2007. His NICU stay was quite a rollercoaster with ups and downs as the NICU life gives you many scares—from brain bleeds, to pneumonia, to worries of blindness, but we kept our faith throughout. In the end, all of his issues were typical preemie issues. He is now three years old and is a living, walking, testament to God's love and everyday miracles. His only complication at this point is that he is asthmatic. He did get RSV when he was 18 months and that caused some damage to his lungs. Asthma is very common in preemies and of all the complications, we'll take that one hands down and with a smile.

While my story is eventful and filled with many complications, I had my post AS miracle thanks be to God and my miracle worker, Dr. March. I had to fight this battle and know I gave it my all. I couldn't give up. I desperately wanted a sibling for my daughter and knew in my heart that God would guide me through this. I hope that my story does give some of you inspiration. Don't let fear affect your decisions. Arm yourself with knowledge and the BEST possible care for your Asherman's. Never lose faith; the doctors will guide you to the best decisions. We are all in this battle together … sisters in our AS struggle and I pray for all our dreams to be realized!! If it wasn't for Poly and my A list doctor, I wouldn't have my baby boy today and for that I am eternally grateful!

16. SUSAN

My Asherman's story begins as so many others, a "simple" medical procedure which affected us so significantly without us even knowing it at the time. My husband and I had some difficulty getting pregnant with our first child. Following oral fertility medications and over a year of trying, we finally conceived and gave birth to a beautiful baby boy. Two weeks later, I began experiencing dark, bloody clots with one the size of a golf ball. I made an appointment with my midwife and she manually removed additional material which she stated was part of my placenta. She scheduled me with a surgeon for a dilation and curettage to remove any remaining placenta. This procedure seemed to be commonplace and in my brief discussions with her and my surgeon only minimal long-term complications were addressed. Asherman's Syndrome was never mentioned. One year later, we decided to attempt conceiving again as we didn't want to delay due to our past fertility issues. I had not menstruated since prior to my first pregnancy but attributed this to the fact I had nursed for a year.

After taking medication in an attempt to jump start my cycle without success, my OB/GYN performed a hysteroscopy to determine if there was a problem. When he initially said Asherman's, describing what it was and what had probably caused it, I felt numb and did not fully comprehend what he was saying. My next thought was that it could be fixed and I assumed it would be a brief delay in our attempts to get pregnant. When he told me I would need to see a specialist, I began to get scared. I had always assumed that having children would come naturally and my husband and I had considered having three to four children despite my previous problems with ovulation. Our physician had no concerns about us conceiving again despite my past fertility issues and the diagnosis of Asherman's was a huge blow.

After having our first child we assumed that the rest may come easier since my body had experienced pregnancy once already. Becoming pregnant and having children had always been a part of my life which I had never questioned.

On the day I was diagnosed with Asherman´s, not only did I question my family's future, but also my identity as a woman. I felt like I failed myself, my husband and my son because I may not be capable of having any more babies. We all picture how our life is going to be and the roles we will play. Our plan had included parenthood and multiple children. It was incredibly depressing knowing that we may never experience this and my own feelings of loss were heightened by the fact that my body's inability to reproduce may deprive my husband of more children and my son of having siblings to grow up with. I knew that adoption was a possibility but this was not a comfort at the time. It felt as though I was letting down my family even though I couldn't have prevented Asherman's. My sister, my friends, other acquaintances seemed to get pregnant and give birth with no difficulties or complications at all. My body was the one that was failing us as a family. I had also linked my personal identity and a part of my being a woman with experiencing pregnancy, childbirth and raising children. Emotionally I felt like less of a woman because of my body's inadequacy. Asherman´s is not a choice like birth control, permanent or otherwise. It took away what should have been my natural ability as a woman to get pregnant and I had difficulty adjusting my perception of myself with this new limitation.

With the diagnosis of Asherman's we went through a gamut of emotions from anger to sadness to feelings of despair. After we did some research and met with the specialist, we felt some hope though I attempted to accept that I may not have any more children even with his assurances. We had multiple procedures to remove the scarring followed by months of fertility treatments including injected medications and insemination. We looked into IVF as well assuming this would be our final alternative but never had to take this step. My lining was very thin following removal of the scarring but the specialist felt we could still conceive. I don't know if anyone can fully understand the frustration and patience that this process requires if they have not been through it themselves. It means taking medications which make you feel ill and driving a distance to the doctor's office morning after morning to have an uncomfortable procedure done. This is followed by more waiting until you can finally take a pregnancy test. Then dealing with the pain and disappointment of a negative test and counting down the days for your period to start so that you can embark on the entire process all over again. Month after month. It was exhausting with months of disappointment and depression.

I felt as though I was in a strange vacuum in which our entire lives were driven by the attempt to conceive. There was an overlying feeling of sadness combined with anticipation and then a feeling of loss with each negative test and menstruation. The added stress of traveling to the doctor's, taking the medications and working full-time did take its toll. We were lucky that my husband is a stay at home dad so he was able to take on some of the household burdens but it was still a tense time. I was blessed with an understanding director and supportive co-workers who allowed me some flexibility with my work schedule. My work was an hour and a half from the doctor's office and I did not always feel very well after the procedures were done. I also struggled talking about this very personal experience as I tended to try putting on a happy face rather than sharing my emotions. It was painful to talk about and challenging to discuss because no one in my immediate circle of friends, family, co-workers had gone through this.

My relationship with my husband was strained during this time as well due to the stress of the situation and because our times of intimacy were affected by where I was in my cycle. It didn't feel natural to attempt this through insemination but it was our best hope to get pregnant. My husband was wonderful during this time despite his own frustration acting as support for myself and caring for our son. My son was too young to fully understand what was going on though he was aware that mommy was tired and feeling unwell at times. I'm certain that he could tell that my husband and I were both emotionally drained even though we attempted to maintain as much normalcy as possible. Overall, it was a difficult time for us as a family and we turned to our faith and family to help sustain us.

In the final month in which we could have an insemination, we decided to use the medications but try to get pregnant without this intervention. We were one of the lucky ones and somehow, miraculously, we were blessed with a pregnancy. The pregnancy itself was unremarkable though I was very fearful at the beginning I may miscarry since my lining was so thin. We also had some bleeding in the early months but without any complications. During the pregnancy, I was more cautious than with my first and nervous overall. Even the smallest thing that seemed out of the ordinary worried me. I saw a specialist for the initial portion of the pregnancy and then was transitioned to a regular obstetrician. In the end I did develop preeclampsia and had to be induced. On Thanksgiving Day 2008, we gave birth to a healthy baby boy.

The effects of Asherman's were present even at his birth. I required an immediate dilation and curettage for another retained placenta. As I was shifted to a different bed for the procedure a large amount of blood flowed out. I began to feel lightheaded and could tell that my blood pressure was dropping. I remember telling this to the nurse and do not remember anything else until I was being transported to ICU. I had hemorrhaged a significant amount of blood and required blood transfusions. As I was headed to the ICU I felt like I was in a haze. I overheard the nurse say "ICU" and feared there was something wrong with our baby. When I questioned her she reassured me that the baby was fine and I was the one being transferred due to my blood loss. It was a strange sense of confused relief to hear this, as I still was not fully cognizant of what was happening.

My husband told me afterward that the doctor had come out of the operating room looking shell shocked. He overheard a nurse saying that she had been called to the floor for an emergency because things had gotten bad in the operating room. Everything happened so quickly they had not told him what exactly was going on. In that moment, he told me that he remembered thinking that he couldn't panic because of our children and wondered how he was going to manage if he had to raise them on his own. It was surreal for both of us, I was too sick to fully understand the seriousness of the situation and I think that my husband was in the mindset that this couldn't be happening to our family. All of our lives could have been drastically altered in that short period of time.

The next day our doctor told us that he had never seen so much blood. They continued to monitor my levels and luckily additional transfusions were not necessary. I felt amazingly better. The next day though, I still had a general feeling of weakness and fatigue. I was able to nurse my baby and care for him with minimal difficulty. We were just so thankful that they had saved my life and for the tiny miracle which had been given to us.

It has been a year since my son's birth and we are all doing fine. I still have not menstruated and I am assuming the Asherman's is present again, though I have not had any tests to confirm this. Our OB/GYN is recommending that we not attempt to have any more children either way due to the hemorrhaging. We have had a mixture of emotions regarding this over the past year. We are sad that we won't be having any more children while at the same time being so very thankful for the two we have. There are times that I think about trying again despite our doctor's warnings and the likelihood we would have to go through all of the surgeries and fertility treatments again. This desire for more children is especially strong as some of my friends have become pregnant again emphasizing our inability. Sometimes I wonder if it may be worth the risk to go through the process again and try for another baby to complete the family we intended to have. In the end I would never want to do something which could risk my life and ultimately hurt my children and our family.

For the most part we are simply thankful and feel fortunate to have our children. Not everyone with Asherman's is so lucky and we are grateful that we were given this gift as many others have tried without success. I empathize with what all of the women are going through in this journey to fight Asherman's in their own individual way. This experience has made me realize how blessed we are and to appreciate both of our children more. It has taught me how amazing the gift of life truly is.

17. LEANNE

The pregnancy that resulted in my now two-year-old daughter was very straightforward and without any complications. She was conceived in the first month that we tried, and everything went very smoothly until her birth. Since I was overdue, I was induced; my waters broke, but I never went in to labor and had to have a Caesarean section. My daughter was born at 6:30 p.m. on September 26, 2007, and she was perfect.

In hindsight, not going in to labor was a good thing, given the problems I had with a deeply attached placenta. The trouble started when the doctor tried to remove it. It was attached very deeply, and in the process of its removal, I lost two liters of blood and I really thought I was going to just close my eyes and never wake up. At one stage, the doctors even talked about removing my uterus, which is not something any woman who wants to have children wants to hear on the operating table. I received a blood transfusion following the Caesarean section and only then began to believe that I was not going to leave my newborn baby without a mother.

Once I had recovered from my daughter's birth I thought all the drama was behind me. However, when my daughter was four weeks old, I started bleeding and my general practitioner (GP) put me on antibiotics. I also had an ultrasound, which showed retained placenta; as a result, my GP referred me to our local specialist OB/GYN, and she removed the remaining placenta via a hysteroscopy. However, she was concerned about the amount of bleeding during the procedure and as well as whether she had in fact removed all of the placenta, which she had literally picked out bit by bit. She mentioned to me the risk of my periods not returning after such an operation due to the walls of the uterus scarring together. I remember feeling very overwhelmed, and I started thinking that my daughter would be an only child; this was really hard to contemplate as I had always wanted two children. I couldn't believe that something like this would happen to me, so after the initial shock wore off, I pushed to the back of my mind the possibility that I might not be able to have another child and went ahead with the removal of the retained placenta. After the procedure to remove it, I concentrated all of my efforts on being a new mum and my worries about having more children faded away.

Since I was breastfeeding my daughter, I wasn't expecting my period to return for some time. However, when she was eight months old I got my first period since her birth. It was different from past periods, though: it was so painful, with less blood, and even that was more brown than red. I put up with the painful periods for about four months before seeing my GP, who recommended a blood test and ultrasound. Both were normal. As I was not trying to conceive another baby at the time, I put my concerns to the back of my head. It couldn't be too bad, I reasoned, as I was having periods, even if they were very different from the pre-baby ones (a lot of books I had read suggested that this could be normal after a pregnancy).

In May 2009 we started trying for another baby. After four months of trying, I was convinced that something was not right with my body, since my daughter was conceived straightaway and it had taken only three months to conceive after a previous miscarriage. The nagging thoughts of not being able to have more children came flooding back so I then turned to the Internet for some information. I found the Asherman's Syndrome website and joined the AS support group, which was just a fabulous resource. I felt like I finally knew what was wrong with me as everything I read about Asherman's Syndrome was exactly what I was experiencing. It seemed I was not alone in diagnosing myself, and in this day and age, I find it bizarre that so many women with AS – instead of the doctors who are meant to be the experts – must do so. I made an appointment with the specialist OB/GYN who had removed the retained placenta, but I had to wait almost three months for the appointment (I live in a city with a population of 30,000 people and only one specialist OB/GYN). In the meantime I read everything I could and decided to e-mail an A-list AS doctor in Australia. He replied very quickly and said it was highly likely that I had AS, and it was such a relief that I didn't have to convince the doctor that something was wrong with me. He could also fit me in pretty much whenever I could organize the trip. So the wheels were set in motion and things moved very quickly. I often questioned myself: Was I doing the right thing by travelling to the other side of the country, especially when I had not actually been diagnosed with Asherman's Syndrome and as such didn't have any concrete evidence that I even had Asherman's Syndrome? I reasoned that I knew something was wrong with me and that even if it wasn't Asherman's Syndrome, the doctor I was travelling to see would know what it was. I also read some information posted on the AS website by another A-list AS doctor, who said, "To hope that my inexperienced local doctor will do the job well is taking a risk. We all travel far distances and spend money for goals less important than good health." I also couldn't put a price on giving my daughter a brother or sister and I didn't want to be wishing that I had gone to see an A-list AS doctor when I had the means available to me, so I flew to Sydney at the end of September 2009 and the doctor did the hysteroscopy the next day, removing all of the scarring. I was diagnosed with stage II Asherman's and was considered a mild case. The scarring was mainly at the cervix and on the right side of my uterus where my daughter's placenta had been attached. I was put on estrogen for twenty-one days and got my period on day 11 of the estrogen; I was advised to stop the estrogen and to start trying to conceive. My first period after my surgery was such a beautiful thing: It was not painful at all, and the blood was so red with no brown blood in sight. I knew I had done the right thing. It is funny how as women we go through most of our lives not looking forward to our period but when you have AS you will do anything to have a normal period.

On the second cycle I became pregnant, and I am now 15 weeks pregnant. I had an ultrasound at six weeks and there was a heartbeat; it was truly amazing as for a while I didn't think I would get the chance to give my daughter a brother or sister. Everything in my pregnancy has been progressing as normally as possible. I will be travelling to Perth next month (which is a four-hour drive from where I live) to have an extensive scan and maybe even an MRI so the doctors can have a good look at the placenta to see if there is any evidence of placenta accreta. Depending on what the scan shows I may have to travel back to Perth for the birth so I can have the baby in a tertiary hospital. I am trying not to get too ahead of myself and also to stop wishing the time away, as I feel like I won't be able to stop worrying that everything is going to be ok with me and my baby until it is finally here safely and in my arms. The whole AS experience has really taught me never to take my fertility for granted ever again. I know it is still in the early days, but we are off to a great start, so I am hoping the next six months pass very uneventfully and the birth even more so.

Thanks to Poly and all of the fantastic ladies who give up so much of their own time to help others – it is truly amazing and we are all so lucky to have the fabulous resource the AS support group provides.

18. LAUREN

My husband and I decided to start a family in the summer of 2004. I found out I was pregnant in October of 2004, but soon learned it was not a viable pregnancy, so I went on to have a dilation and curettage (D&C). I thought it would be a simple procedure, one that would allow me to quickly get past my loss, and move on to trying to conceive again. I was not offered an alternate solution and I was not advised of any risks with this procedure. I had problems with bleeding after the dilation and curettage; several weeks went by and it did not stop. I had to be dilated in my doctor's office and she performed a suction to remove some "product" that was left in my uterus. This was more unpleasant than the actual dilation and curettage as I was awake and scared. Again, I was not warned of any risks or given any alternate solutions. The bleeding finally stopped several days after the procedure.

I fell pregnant again in January 2005 but at an 8-week-ultrasound, my doctor could not detect a heartbeat. She sent me to a radiologist for a second opinion. The radiologist confirmed that there was no heartbeat and also gave me more bad news. There was a second fetus, also with no heartbeat. This was much more devastating and harder news for me to digest. I wondered why this was happening to me and my doctor could not provide answers. It was summed up to be bad luck. I went on to have my second D&C in March 2005. Again I was not offered any alternate solutions and I was not advised of any risks. Again I had bleeding problems after the second D&C. In April 2005, I began to hemorrhage, my obstetrician at the time believed I may have had a molar pregnancy. Due to the amount of bleeding and fear of infection I was admitted to the hospital immediately for my third D&C. This time I was advised by my doctor that if she could not control the bleeding I would need a hysterectomy. At this point I was numb yet nervous. I didn't know how to make sense of all of this in my mind. I kept asking myself over and over, "how can having a baby be so difficult?" It seemed as though everyone around me was having a baby. But I had no answer so I remained numb. I cringed when people would ask me, "when are you going to start a family?" I would come up with smart answers for them saying things like "I don't want to get fat". I began looking into adoption and discovered very quickly how expensive it was. We could certainly never afford it.

After the third D&C I was put on birth control pills and had blood drawn every month for six months to make sure the pregnancy hormone returned to zero and stayed at zero. In January 2006, per the recommendation from my obstetrician, I began seeing a reproductive endocrinologist (RE), a specialist in reproductive medicine. He ran blood tests, and performed a hysterosalpingogram (HSG), an X-ray of the uterus and fallopian tubes which allows visualization of the inside of the uterus and tubes. The picture will reveal any abnormalities of the uterus as well as tubal problems such as blockage and dilation. I met with him in his office to discuss the results of the HSG. When he showed me the X-Ray results, he pointed to a large area and told me he didn't know if it was scar tissue or if I had a congenital abnormality like a septum. He wouldn't know for certain what was happening inside my uterus until he went "inside it". I remember being completely freaked out as he explained this to me. I remember breaking down as soon as I got into my car in the parking lot. I cried for what seemed like hours. I was so scared. All I kept thinking was that I must be some kind of freak of nature and I was afraid of what my husband would think. Would he want to stay with me if I had an abnormality and couldn't have his children? It was a dark day and I remember it vividly. It still brings back bad feelings.

In May 2006 my RE performed a laparoscopy and a hysteroscopy. I was diagnosed with a severe case of Asherman's Syndrome. He told me it was very difficult to remove as the scar tissue was very dense. I woke up with a balloon in my uterus to keep the sides from adhering together and I was given a prescription for 30 days of estrogen and seven days of progesterone. I started researching Asherman's Syndrome; I was very upset with all the information I found. My hope of having a baby was diminished.

In August 2006 my RE performed a second HSG to see what my uterus looked like after the surgery and see if the scarring was gone. He told me while I was still on the X-ray table that things looked much better and that he was pleased with the condition of my uterus. He told me to call his office and make an appointment with my husband to discuss the results in more detail. I was so nervous going into that appointment that I was sick to my stomach. When we met with him, he showed us the video from the camera used during the surgery. And he told us we could immediately start trying to conceive. I was thrilled, relieved, and nervous all at the same time.

We began trying right away. One of my girlfriends gave me a digital ovulation monitor so we could take the guess work out of it. Four long months went by. I couldn't understand why I wasn't getting pregnant, it had happened so easily in the past and now we had the help of a digital monitor … I became very emotional. I wondered if something else was wrong with me. All the baggage from my past was obviously still with me. But, happily, I discovered I was pregnant in December 2006. The happiness of the pregnancy was quickly replaced by constant worry. I bled during the first three months of my pregnancy, quite heavy at times. I was never given a reason why other than I have a "lousy" uterus. During the first trimester, I went to my RE every week for an ultrasound. This was my RE's normal course of action for his newly pregnant patients. Each week was full of mixed emotions. I made myself sick with worry before each ultrasound. Thinking for certain that it would be the week I lost the baby. But, each week, it was positive news. My RE released me to my obstetrician's care. I switched to a new obstetrician so I was no longer seeing the doctor who caused my Asherman's. After researching Asherman's Syndrome, I couldn't ever bring myself to go back to her. I was confused with how I felt about her, and after what she did to me, in the way she altered my life, I didn't trust her medically.

Each visit to the doctor was positive. I could not, however, allow myself to enjoy my first successful pregnancy. I was certain that something would go wrong. The thought of losing another baby was unimaginable, and I still kept expecting the worst. I would get very worried if I didn't feel the baby moving enough. I even rented a fetal Doppler so I could hear the baby's heartbeat when I was uncertain. The worst, however, did not happen. I delivered my son, James, via C-section due to fetal distress during labor, on August 16th, 2007. I had bleeding problems after the birth of James. I was told after a C-section that my bleeding should be light and for a short duration. It seemed to finally slow down after five weeks, but then picked up again and was very heavy after six weeks postpartum. I pressed at one of the doctor's in the practice, not my main doctor, that something was wrong. The doctor finally ordered an ultrasound which revealed retained placenta.

It was a Friday morning when she called me with the results of the retained placenta. She told me that it was a very small piece. She also told me that after delivery, often small pieces of the placenta get left behind, and the uterus will normally pass them. But since I have Asherman's Syndrome the inside of my uterus is very "tacky" making my uterus unable to expel it. She wanted to schedule a D&C for Monday. I was surprised at how quickly they wanted to do it and I demanded she contact my RE for guidance. She did speak with him and informed me that either she, or my main doctor who performed the delivery, would be doing the D&C under ultrasound guidance. I was happy with the decision, as I knew I faced problems with infection if I did not have the retained placenta removed, but I was still worried about what it would mean for my future and the possibilities of having another baby. My main obstetrician called to tell me he would be performing the surgery himself. He came to speak with me the morning of the surgery, after I was already admitted, and told me that based on my history he decided he was going to do a hysteroscopy instead of the D&C. I was so relieved that I almost hugged him. The surgery was successful and the bleeding stopped.

I went back to my RE in February 2008. I wanted to make sure that my Asherman's had not returned, and if it did, I wanted to deal with it immediately. He performed another HSG, and to my surprise, there was little scarring. He explained that sometimes a healthy pregnancy can help restore and heal a uterus. He told me that I could start trying to conceive whenever I was ready. In April 2008 I stopped taking my birth control pills and my menstrual periods resumed to "normal" almost immediately.

I discovered I was pregnant with my second post-Asherman's baby in July 2008. It was an eventful pregnancy, which was upsetting as I never had time to enjoy the first pregnancy. I had promised myself that if I ever did get pregnant again, I would worry less, and I would try to enjoy it. But again, I was gypped. I would not get to enjoy this pregnancy either, for much different reasons. The bleeding began days after the positive home pregnancy test. Again I had weekly sonograms at my RE's office. In the beginning they were not going well. I remember on a Thursday morning, in my sixth week, my RE told me that he thought I had a blighted ovum, which would explain the bleeding. He scheduled me for another sonogram on

Monday morning. I was numb that Monday morning. I was hoping that the fetus had passed and I would not need another surgery. However, to my surprise we saw a heartbeat. My RE said the fetus had "rallied". My rollercoaster ride of a pregnancy began. The bleeding continued throughout my first trimester. There were times that I bled heavy enough to soak through a pad in less than an hour. I had two subchorionic hematomas, which caused most of the bleeding. I was on bed rest from week 6 to 14. It was also determined at 12 weeks that my cervix was shortening so I had a cerclage placed at 14 weeks. After the cerclage I was allowed to resume my normal daily activities. At 23 weeks, however, I was admitted to the hospital for pre-term labor. Fortunately, the doctors were able to stop the labor using multiple shots of terbutaline. I was released from the hospital after four days when I begged my doctor to let me go home, promising that I would do anything he told me I needed to do. I was placed on bed rest at home for the remainder of the pregnancy. It was a very scary time. My doctor told me that I had to make it at least another five weeks in order to have a real chance at a positive outcome; fortunately I made it longer than the five weeks. It was also a very difficult time. I had a 17 month old son at home who could not understand why his Mommy couldn't play with him, bathe him, change his diaper, etc. But we managed to find ways to make it work.

Still, the rollercoaster continued. At a 32 week sonogram (I was having them weekly) I was diagnosed with possible placenta increta which an MRI confirmed. Due to the complications increta can cause, we started to plan the delivery. I was scheduled to have an amniocentesis at 37 weeks to confirm the baby's lung maturity. I was to be delivered in the hospital's main operating room that Monday, three days after the amniocentesis. This was necessary because of the potential blood loss an increta can cause.

At 35 weeks, however, I went into labor on my own. I hadn't been feeling well all day, and I thought I had a stomach virus. I called my doctor because something didn't "feel right". With my history, he asked me to come to the hospital to be on the safe side. The contractions started in the car ride to the hospital and they moved quickly. They were less than two minutes apart by the time my husband and I arrived at the hospital. They tried to stop the contractions again. They tried three different medications, but could not stop them. I remember the doctor on call sitting down next to me and very calmly telling me that I was having the baby within the hour. They were prepping the main operating room. They were having blood delivered in case I needed a transfusion, and they were having a bladder specialist there too because they weren't sure how far the increta had grown and I may need to have bladder reconstructive surgery. I also learned right then that I would be receiving a vertical incision for my C-section. It was too much to absorb and everything was moving quickly. The on call doctor contacted my main doctor and he came to perform the delivery. The delivery was hard and it took them close to three hours from start to finish. They put me unconscious after I saw my son, Eamon, on March 9th, 2009.

While I was pregnant with Eamon, my husband and I decided that it was best for me to have a tubal ligation. We could simply not risk another pregnancy or the potential problems it could cause me, or a future baby. Since we knew I was having a C-section, it would be easiest to have it done at the time of the birth. My doctors concurred with the request, and while they do not usually recommend it, encouraged me, due to my history and current circumstances, that it was the right decision. I am extremely lucky to have two beautiful children. I know how fortunate I am. There are many women who do not get to have one baby after being diagnosed with Asherman's, let alone two. Yet, I cannot help but feel that my decision to have the tubal ligation, was determined by Asherman's, and its complications, rather than by what I truly wanted. It was a difficult journey, and I still have residual Asherman's related problems, filled with many tears, much emotional pain, a lot of worry, and constant self-doubt. One I would do again without hesitation or question. There were many times I wanted to give up. I cannot count the number of times I felt inept as a woman and as a wife or how many times I cried. It was a dark time. Somehow, I managed to persevere and push forward. I discovered an inner strength that I did not think I had. The journey can be a long and difficult one, but with faith and hope and the right doctor's care, this Syndrome can be beat.

19. LAURA

In June of 2006, after being married for three years and having just finished painting every room in our new home, we were ready to take the leap into parenthood. Being a parent was always something I had dreamed about. Growing up as an only child I longed for a big family. I knew logically that sometimes it could take a while and things happened but still somehow I thought that wouldn't be me. We proceeded with the carefree attitude of we would not actively "try" but not do anything to prevent it either.

One month later, after being away for the July 4th weekend, I realized that I was late and I took a test after work. I couldn't believe how quick the pink lines appeared. I quickly ripped into the digital test and took that one too and jumped up and down as the word pregnant appeared. I giddily waited for my husband to get home from work like a kid with an A paper to show dad and as soon as he walked in the door I greeted him by telling him he was going to be a daddy! I still remember to this day what a jubilant moment that was.

We went for our first appointment with my doctor around 7 weeks and we were able to see the heartbeat fluttering. The "little bean" as we would call it was so small yet already held all our hope and dreams. I remember walking out of the office on a cloud with our ultrasound picture clutched in my hands. Again we knew that things could happen but we felt confident after seeing the little bean's heartbeat and so we shared the news by presenting the framed sonogram to our family at dinner.

Our first hiccup happened when we traveled to Oregon for a wedding and on our layover on the way, I started spotting. Panic seized me in the bathroom and I thought I would be sick. From long distance, the doctor assured us that this can be normal and to take it easy. We decided not to mention anything to anyone at the wedding and we did our best to just put on a happy face and try to be in the moment. From the airport back home in New York, we traveled directly to the doctor's office where we waited four hours before I was seen. The ultrasound showed again a strong heartbeat and a bigger baby. Relief flooded us and we felt like we had made it to the other side. Again we left on a cloud of happiness mixed with pure exhaustion. At this appointment, my doctor informed us that she no longer delivers and I would have to find a new doctor. No problem, she could have told me anything at this point I was just too elated to care. Fast forward a few weeks later and we go to see our new local OB for the first time. I was 11 weeks at this point and had had no other spotting or issues to speak of. We waited till the typical 12-week-mark to share the news with our colleagues but most friends and family already knew. I remember being in such a blissful dreamy state, what will the baby be, what name will we pick, who will he or she resemble and the ever important what stroller will I register for. These were the things that flooded my consciousness.

We waited in the room and I was just so excited to see the baby again and maybe hear the heartbeat this time but the minute the doctor started I knew something was wrong. He would not meet my eyes and just stared at the screen with the most serious face I had seen. I am sure this must be one of the harder parts of his job so usually full of bringing in life to the world to have to let someone know the baby is gone. "I am so sorry" he uttered "but there is no heartbeat". Complete numbness filled me, I remember looking over to my husband and scanning his face and sadly only seeing the same thing. Completely lost and confused the doctor explained that these things happen, the good news was we got pregnant quickly, it would happen again for us soon is what he said. More sad faces on the way out the door and we left with a follow-up sonogram and a scheduled surgery for a D&C the next day. The smallest glimmer of hope remained that somehow the doctor was wrong but at the later sonogram, the loss was confirmed and so we headed to the hospital. There was no discussion of any other option besides a D&C and at this point I remember feeling anxious to be able to move on with life. The feeling of being pregnant but with a baby that is no longer there is absolutely devastating.

My memory of getting to the hospital is a blur, I remember nurses greeting us and squeezing my hand and handing over tissues and sitting in the gown waiting in the small room with my husband. I remember escorting into the operating room with all of the bright lights and it being so cold and of course them asking me to count backwards and then it was all over and we were back home. Comfort from friends and family flooded in and I was amazed at how many people had miscarriages that I had never known. It was like I was part of some inner circle now and I was very much not alone. We would get through this and we would move on to have our family I felt sure of it.

This was how our story into the world of infertility started. I felt confident that this would be our only hiccup and we would quickly join the ranks of parents like all of our friends before us. However, for us our story took a few more bumps and turns.

We went on to have three more miscarriages after this first one. During this time we saw numerous doctors and underwent many tests to try and identify what might be causing these losses. I mentioned feeling part of an inner circle after our first loss where people understood what you were going through, but as the losses continued the circle we belonged to got smaller and smaller to where we felt like we were standing all by ourselves. The happy ending stories diminished and people started asking us if we had considered adoption and maybe this was just not meant to be. People looked and acted towards me differently, no one knew what to say and the pity was so transparent it hurt to be around others. It was like with each miscarriage we went into a smaller pot, a statistical minority. It felt as if we were now completely and utterly alone in our circumstance.

What kept me going was the pure drive to figure this out. I refused to accept that we would not be parents somehow. I quickly found out that we did not fit into any clean cut "category". The doctors for the most part were encouraged by our ease of getting pregnant and told us it was just "bad luck" and eventually one would stick; it seemed like no one really knew what to tell us. Even the insurance company was not clear what to do with us. I had to fight like crazy for them to approve certain tests and procedures. Only days after my third loss I was on the phone and an insurance agent told me that they would not approve the test because I did not fit in the category of "infertility", after all I was "successfully getting pregnant" as she put it. While she had to wait for me to stop sobbing to answer I declared that to me "successfully" would mean carrying the baby to term. A few managers later I had approval but was confronted with this discrepancy a few more times during our journey.

The second and third miscarriages were early on and so I went through them at home and did not need surgery. The fourth miscarriage we had made it to 12 weeks. The doctor had been watching me very closely and we were able to see the baby grow and hear the heartbeat every week at our sonograms. I remember the appointment day so clearly, it was probably the first appointment that we were more relaxed and I think we felt we had overcome some hurdles. At the previous sonogram the doctor had commented that this one "was a keeper" and we had watched the baby flip over. Usually at the appointments we were silent until the doctor started and then announced loudly "I see a heartbeat"! This appointment again was different and we were joking and talking while he got ready. I will never forget the deafening silence that filled the room as he started the sonogram that day and he did not have to say anything to me. I immediately threw my hands over my face in disbelief and just uttered the word "No", over and over again. Like a two-year-old having a tantrum I just could not let the reality sink in. My husband tried to console me but I was in a dense fog. Again I numbly listened as we prepared for the follow-up sonogram and the D&C. I remember my doctor holding my hand and talking to us but I could not tell you anything that he said.

After this loss and second D&C, I noticed that my period was not coming. I felt all the symptoms of a period, cramping, etc. and I would rush to check but nothing. I called my OB and he told me that my body had been through an awful lot and it would just take time. After another month I called again and this time they gave me medicine to help my period come and still I felt the cyclical cramping but still nothing. I said to my doctor it seems like I am having my period but it is just not able to come out. I went in for a sonogram and the doctor could not see any blockages or anything out of the ordinary. Again I was told just to be patient and it will come.

This was not really my nature and so off to the Internet I went which of course are both a blessing and a curse. I did a quick search on my symptoms and promptly freaked out about possibly having a myriad of diseases. Upon reading further the one that stuck with me was something called Asherman´s Syndrome. I asked my OB about it and he said that it is very rare and only occurs in a small percentage of cases. Well at this point I certainty felt like if anyone would be in the small percentage cases it was me. I found the Asherman´s Yahoo Group, which was an enormous wealth of information as well as a great support system for women going through this not so rare condition, as I found out. After researching for specialists, I found a doctor in our area who received an A rating from the group, I immediately made an appointment with him and after a somewhat painful procedure we learned that unfortunately my hunch was correct and my lower uterus was scarred completely shut. Initially I felt relief that we had a diagnosis but that of course was quickly replaced by just feeling completely overwhelmed. How many more hurdles would we be faced with? We were already facing an uphill battle and now here was another issue, which gave us some hope but no guarantee. I questioned if we would ever be able to have children.

The only thing I knew how to do was move forward and throw myself into this latest "battle". As I prepared for surgery I read as much as I could about Asherman´s and what would be the best way to prevent my body from re-scarring. I remember having the imagery of all this backed up blood just swishing around in me and I was afraid to run or do anything physical. The doctor explained that we caught it very early and the body has a way of absorbing this back but I just could not shake that image.

I was very anxious for this surgery because there were still so many unknowns. So much of it the surgeon had left to "well, we will see when we get in there", so I was both anxious and scared to wake up and receive the news. After the surgery, I was told that he was able to clear out all of the scarring and put in the balloon to help keep everything open while it healed. We were told that I had a very small uterus and he had to use the smallest balloon they make. This statement would cause me tremendous stress later in my next pregnancy as our baby grew and I worried that my uterus was too small and the poor thing was being smooshed in by my teeny tiny walls but I digress. So we left the hospital with my fixed uterus and my tiny balloon to heal and relax, or so I thought.

Before the surgery they give you an antibiotic to help fight off infection. Mine made me sick, so they switched me to a different type.

During the surgery they also give you an antibiotic intravenously. Well, after a few days home I developed a fever and could not keep anything down. It was pure misery. I was sick from both ends and could do nothing but cry and lay on the bathroom floor. We went in to the doctor where they removed the balloon fearing I was fighting an infection but that didn't help. Finally my amazing husband took charge and said enough is enough and took me to the ER where after two days of being violently ill, I was so weak I could barely walk myself. Turned out I had c-difficile, a rare complication from the antibiotic. Ah yes, the statistical minority struck again, I should have known. The very elementary summary that I understood is that our body houses good and bad bacteria in our gastrointestinal track and sometimes with antibiotics all the good bacteria gets killed off too and then we can become sick.

While relieved to be feeling better, part of me then started worrying about the possibility of re-scarring as the balloon was only in for less than a week and not for two weeks as planned. There was nothing we could do but wait. In my head I had already started thinking about the next surgery and while I would continue to work on this issue, I also was ready to move forward in other ways. My husband and I had gone to numerous adoption information sessions, both international and domestic and during this time we made a step and met with an adoption attorney to see about moving forward that way.

In the two years that had passed I felt like I had mourned the idea that I had always had in my head about being pregnant, or how we would have a family. There was a Dixie chick's song I heard during this time that made me pull over to the side of the road and sob because it spoke so perfectly to how I was feeling at that time. Our whole life we think that when the time comes this is what my body will do and when it fails you, you can't help but feel like less of a woman somehow. My husband did everything he could to make me feel otherwise but I felt like I was letting him down somehow and that was the hardest thing for me to deal with. In my head I knew none of this was the case but still this is hard to not dwell on.

When we started exploring adoption I felt for the first time in a while, hopeful. Listening to people's stories about how they grew their families this way inspired me and my daydreams starting changing from being pregnant to getting a call from a birth mom and flying somewhere to pick up our new child. I felt like becoming parents would happen for us just maybe not the way we always thought. So here I was waiting in the surgeon's office while he did the procedure to be able to look and see the uterus. In my head though I was already thinking that he would tell me he was sorry but it did not look good and I was in the small minority that this happened to, and all the other negative things. Well imagine my surprise when we left that day with an A+ for my uterus and the green light to start trying again. Now what do we do? I was so consumed on just getting myself "fixed" that we never thought of trying to get pregnant again and what did that even include at this point?

My husband and I felt that we had it in us to give pregnancy one more try. We didn't want to take any chances, so we tried all the treatments that were supposed to help and we once again were lucky to get pregnant right away and then the waiting game began. Our first beta was strong, the second doubled, we were cautiously hopeful and then on a Friday afternoon at work I got the call that our betas dropped and it looked like we were losing this pregnancy. We were told to go off all of the medicine and just wait for it to happen naturally. I remember thinking at least it was early and I won't need another surgery.

The very next day we were in a dog store with puppies surrounding us and a little silver dapple Doxie crawled up into my lap and looked into my eyes. That was it, I was smitten. We had our first baby, a little puppy to love and care for. We paid for her and were given all of the instructions on how to care for her and they came out with her wrapped in a little baby blanket. I could not stop the tears from falling as she approached. Of course they could have no idea what was happening for us at that moment and what the significance of that blanket meant. It was not how I imagined having my first baby but instantaneously I was filled with love and she helped ease the pain enormously. I was so genuinely happy in that moment, that my husband later looked back at those photos and commented that Fiona helped bring the light back in my eyes.

The next few days were filled with crate and potty training and of course lots of snuggles and while the loss was still very much on my mind, the new puppy helped dull the pain. By midweek, I was having no signs of a miscarriage I called the doctor and went in for more blood work. I was sure they would have to give me some medicine to bring things on and I remember hoping everything would just happen quickly. That limbo period was always the worst for me. Never did I imagine I would get the call that I did the next day telling us somehow, miraculously, my numbers were not only back up but they were back where they should be for this time. I was stunned and the only thing I could utter was "but we just bought a dog". Why those were my first words, I don't know but I was just in such disbelief. The doctor said in all of his years he had only had this happen once before. Finally we were on the good side of a small statistic.

I was ecstatic but obviously still very cautious and I think that would describe our whole pregnancy. We continued to go weekly for sonograms and as we passed new milestones we got more and more hopeful but never did I take for granted that it could all be taken away.

Once I was able to feel the baby move around inside it was so amazing and such a wonderful reassurance that the baby was growing and striving but on days when things were more still, it took everything in me not to panic and drive to the ER. Luckily for me I had a very active baby. I wish I could say I finally was able to just let go and enjoy the pregnancy but after the losses I did not trust my body fully. While I loved being pregnant it was as if I could not wait for the baby to be born so he or she would be safe from the perils that surely lay within, little did I know once they are born there is much more to worry about.

Then one early morning at 34 weeks my water broke and we headed to the hospital. Many hours later, our little boy was born, small at 5lbs and 3 ounces but perfectly healthy! We had not found out the gender ahead of time, which as you can imagine was a challenge with all of the sonograms that we had, but I would not change that decision for anything because the moment when my husband got to tell me what the baby was, is hands down one of the best moments in my life, along with seeing and holding him of course!

If you had asked me years ago, this is certainly not the path that I would have chosen to have our family but having gone through it, I now realize that this journey made us the people we are today. It strengthened our marriage in ways we never could have imagined and showed us courage within ourselves that we did not even know existed. I am not a particularly religious person but when I look at our son I see this little miracle, a fighter that somehow beat all the odds and thrived to join our family. He is such a happy little kid and his smile lights up my heart and makes me glad every single second of the day that we never gave up on our journey.

20. ANDREA

My story starts in January 2005, when my doctor at the time found a fibroid in my fundus and decided to perform a very aggressive surgery to remove it. I had had three miscarriages to date, and my doctor believed that the fibroid may have been the reason I had miscarried so many times. However, he told me after the surgery that he hadn't been able to find the fibroid but had done some scraping to clear out the last miscarriage. He then suggested I seek another opinion on the potential cause of the miscarriages but also suggested that I try again to conceive: "Maybe it was just bad luck," is what he said. I am thankful we did not take his advice.

I was referred to a reproductive center in Long Beach, and it was there, on March 14, 2005, that I was diagnosed with Asherman's Syndrome. The doctors at the center were alerted to the possibility of Asherman's Syndrome when they learned that my period had never returned post-surgery. Following my diagnosis, I called the office of my previous doctor to let them know that I had Asherman's Syndrome. What was very unfortunate and surprising was that they had never heard of this condition, and that concerned me.

I wondered how this had happened to me and started to research what I was being told I had. To my dismay I found out that Asherman's Syndrome can be caused by severe trauma to the uterus via surgery or an aggressive D&C. I had never been told this was a side effect of an aggressive surgery or a D&C – a procedure that had, in fact, scarred shut my uterus. Several ultrasounds revealed that the back and front walls were stuck together.

The Long Beach reproductive center was not a member of the medical group I originally used, so before my initial visit to the center, I had changed to the group to which it did belong so that my insurance would help pay for the services. After my diagnosis, though, I decided to find the *best* doctor in California to help me, and I did. Unfortunately, my insurance did not cover his services, but we decided it was worth it and that we would pay ourselves for treatment with him.

I had a laparoscopy/hysteroscopy on April 14th to remove the scar tissue from my uterus. Fortunately this surgery was a success; my tubes were clear and the scarring was gone. The bad news came when I found out that the back wall of my uterus was terribly thin due to scraping from a resectoscope. A resectoscope is the tool that was used to scrape away the remains of my last miscarriage. I was told that if that back wall showed thin on my next ultrasound on June 16th, I would not be able to carry my own child and I would need to think of an alternative method of having the one thing that I have wanted with all of my heart!

The fortunate part of this story is that the back wall looked fine when I went for my ultrasound, and on August 3rd, 2005, our doctor gave us the green light to try to conceive. As I had had severe Asherman's, it was truly a miracle. With one operative laparoscopy/hysteroscopy following a failed hysterosalpingogram my scarring was gone, and we got our fertility back after progesterone and estrogen treatments were completed.

This experience was an incredibly difficult time for me and for my family. It took its toll on my husband and our immediate family. It also left me with a lack of trust for the medical community that I did not have before. I am of the mindset now that if I can educate others about this diagnosis, I will do so, if only to keep just one woman from experiencing what I have.

After one ultrasound and a failed HSG I was told by my most recent physician that I had less than a 50/50 chance of ever being able to carry my own child. I was terrified. I wanted to reach out to the former doctor and ask,

"Why would you have been so aggressive on a woman who you knew wanted children?" But I could not bring myself to do this.

I was angry that Asherman's was never mentioned to me. I feel that medical professionals have a duty to inform and educate their patients, and I feel that I was not given that information. I wanted to be a mother, more than any other thing I had ever done in my life. As a woman, having lost my ability to have a child was devastating. I was told that to be parents, we might need to pursue surrogacy or adoption, both of which were incredibly expensive.

The best news out of all of this is that we were able to get pregnant by August 31st, 2005, and my beautiful daughter was born on April 19th, 2006. Shayna was 5 weeks early -- weighing in at 4lbs 8oz -- but healthy!

We will never forget the heartache we experienced through this whole ordeal, but give thanks every day that we were blessed with our daughter. We chose not to have another child for fear of having to go through it again. I am now 42 years old, and my daughter is 2½. I would not change a thing but hope that my story helps others and gives them the power of knowledge.

21. KARINA

My Asherman's Syndrome journey began with a good event. It took us a year to conceive our first son, but my pregnancy was easy and the induction delivery went well. After the delivery, however, I just didn't seem to be healing. I had intense pressure every time I stood for longer than five minutes, even at three weeks postpartum. At three weeks and three days after my son's birth, I started hemorrhaging. I had a D&C the next day for retained products of conception. My local OB performed the procedure, and she told me there was a piece of placenta that was "hanging out" in my cervix, causing it to stay dilated. This explained my pain and pressure sensations. I bled so heavily in the recovery room that I remember the doctor saying, "If she doesn't stop bleeding soon, we'll have to take her back into the OR and do another D&C." I finally stopped bleeding, and after the surgery, it seemed I was on the road to recovery.

I breastfed my son until he was six months old. When he was weaned, I kept expecting my period to return, but at ten months postpartum I still had not had a period. I did notice, however, that I was having a tiny amount of spotting and intense cramping at the time my period should have been coming. I was charting my cycle as well, and I also noticed that I was ovulating. I called my OB at ten months postpartum to report my concerns, but I was told to call back in two months if I still had not gotten my period. After my periods still did not resume, I called back two months later, and my doctor offered me Clomid, since we were planning on trying to conceive again. I was shocked to be offered fertility drugs, since I still had not had a period and it was not clear why. I declined the Clomid and requested an appointment with the doctor to be checked out. At my appointment, I was given an ultrasound and told I had "cervical stenosis". There were visible "pockets of fluid" in my uterus, which were assumed to be trapped blood.

My OB attempted to dilate my cervix, with no anesthesia, in her office. It was extremely painful and unsuccessful. I was scheduled for a cervical dilation under anesthesia. My doctor performed it and told me, "I cleaned out the cervix really well. You should be getting your period soon." I never resumed a period, but I did have the cyclical pain the next cycle, just as before the procedure. I then decided my OB did not know what she was doing with me, and I transferred to a local reproductive endocrinologist. On my initial visit with him, the RE was somewhat skeptical that I had Asherman's Syndrome. I had researched my symptoms online, though, and I knew that this was what I had. He performed an ultrasound, noting the trapped areas of blood, and he admitted I was probably correct. He scheduled me for my first laparoscopy/ hysteroscopy the following month.

During my surgery, the doctor, upon entering the uterus, realized he was visualizing my right fallopian tube from inside the uterus. During my cervical dilation procedure the previous month, my local OB had punctured the uterine wall and pulled the tube back through the opening. It had "healed" that way and had to be dissected out of the wall of the uterus. The procedure, which was supposed to take an hour and a half, ended up taking five and a half hours. After the surgery, I awoke to the news that I had lost a tube and had gone only from 90% scarring to 60% scarring in the uterine cavity. My remaining tube was completely scarred over, and the surgeon said he could not even tell where the tube was supposed to be. He had done his best, but he told us that we would only have another child through adoption or surrogacy. We were devastated. This was just not the news we were expecting. I had thought I would wake up from surgery and be told that I was now free to try to conceive our next child.

One of the worst things for me was the frustration I felt about my initial OB/GYN. At no point, as I was describing my symptoms, had she mentioned Asherman's Syndrome. It frustrated me to know that I had been able to diagnose myself just from doing a quick search on the Internet, but my trusted doctor seemed unaware of Asherman's Syndrome being a risk of the D&C, a procedure she was performing frequently.

Once I got my wits back about me, I began communicating with the ladies in the group from ashermans.org and decided to contact one of the A-list doctors recommended by the group. After a phone consult with him, I made the decision to fly across the country to have surgery with him. He was able to completely remove my scarring and determined that the left tube was open. After the post-op hormones and weekly cervical dilations he recommended, I had an HSG and saw that I still had about 30% scarring remaining. I flew out to see the A-lister again for surgery. This time, the follow-up HSG showed about 25% scarring remaining. The doctor felt he had done all he could and gave us the green light to try to conceive, with the understanding that early miscarriages were a real possibility.

I got pregnant the first month we tried, but I lost that pregnancy at 4 weeks, 3 days. I got pregnant again the next month. Despite heavy bleeding for twelve weeks, I managed to hold on to the pregnancy. I had concerns about cervical issues, due to my many dilations, so I requested a preventative cerclage at 12 weeks. The cerclage was placed, which was a real blessing since my OB could see alarming cervical changes as early as 14 weeks. I began contracting at 16 weeks, and at 19 weeks began 17p injections, which are progesterone shots used to prevent preterm contractions and labor. I had a very short cervix by 27 weeks, and I was put on bed rest. Amazingly, I made it to 37 weeks, when I had a scheduled C-section, per order of the A-list doctor.

My delivery was uncomplicated. My OB said there was one small area that was "a little stuck" to the uterine wall, but the placenta came out with no real problems. My son weighed 5lb., 15 oz., and is healthy and beautiful, and we feel that he is a true miracle. We are a very spiritual family and give God all of the credit for bringing this little boy to us. My personal belief, though, is that He worked his miracle through the amazing hands of the very skilled A-list surgeon we found through the Asherman's support group. The ladies in the group were so helpful, and always willing to answer questions and calm my fears.

22. KATHY

YEAR ONE: TRYING TO CONCEIVE

My particular story takes place over a five-year period, and it started in the summer of 2001. My husband and I had been married for a happy five years, and our next step in life was to start our family. I was 31 at the time, and my husband was five years younger, at 26. For several months we talked about when I should go off the pill, as we were both scared to be parents, as well as excited. I went off the pill during the summer and expected to be pregnant within a few months. Wow, was I wrong! I would never have believed it if someone told me ahead of time that I'd have to endure a misdiagnosis, a punctured uterus, multiple unnecessary medications, way too many surgeries, a miscarriage, and years of heartbreak and frustration before becoming a parent.

In the beginning, trying to get pregnant was a fun and exciting thing. Each month I thought, "This is it, I'm pregnant!" yet each month my period came right on time. I started buying ovulation kits that confirmed I was ovulating each month, and we made sure our timing was perfect, but the pregnancy tests were still negative. As the months went by, things started to get frustrating; after all, every one of our friends got pregnant right away, so why couldn't it happen for us? We also met people along the way who got pregnant even when they didn't want to … talk about frustrating!

YEAR TWO: MISDIAGNOSIS

After an entire year of trying, we decided to go to a reproductive endocrinologist (RE). My OB/GYN doctor, who, herself, was a wonderful woman that suffered infertility and was never able to have children of her own (yet brought babies into the world every day), referred me to a specialist. Little did I know at the time, but this specialist would misdiagnose me, puncture my uterus, perform an unsuccessful laparoscopy, and have me on a multitude of unnecessary hormones. Of course, at the time, I thought to myself, "Ok, this will be easy, the doctor will fix me and I'll be pregnant in no time." Wrong again!

I was a nervous wreck going to my first RE visit. I had no idea what to expect, didn't know much about the ins and outs of getting pregnant (aside from the sex part!), and just really felt weird about talking to a stranger about how I wasn't able to get pregnant. Thankfully, my husband went with me and shared the same trepidation as I did. As we sat through the one hour consultation, answering all sorts of embarrassing questions (sexual history, boxers or briefs, etc.), we came out of the meeting feeling a new sense of hope that things would be going our way soon. And yes, once again I was wrong!

My baseline blood tests all came back normal and my first vaginal ultrasound was normal as well. The RE decided to try me on a Clomid challenge test to help shorten my cycle length (they ranged around 35 to 45 days) along with ultrasound monitoring, a semen analysis, and a hysterosalpingogram (HSG). When my husband's semen analysis came back perfectly healthy, he was gleaming (especially after the RE let him see them swimming under a microscope.) I, on the other hand, didn't have the same reaction. Yes, I was happy that he didn't have any problems, but that pretty much meant that the problem was with me, and I felt a lot of guilt and sadness over that fact.

On the day of the HSG exam, I was a nervous wreck. I already suffer from generalized anxiety, and going into unfamiliar situations really tend to kick my anxiety up a notch. My husband went with me and was able to watch the exam in the x-ray room with me. At the time, no one (including myself) knew that I had extensive adhesions throughout 90% of my uterus. The RE tried his best to insert the scope up into my uterus without success. The exam was excruciating for me and I was crying on the x-ray table as the doctor was trying to insert the scope. My husband felt so helpless watching me in so much pain and not being able to do anything about it. As the RE kept pushing at the scope, he eventually broke through some of my adhesions, but he was pushing so hard that the scope punctured my uterus and the exam had to be immediately cancelled. The doctor told me to go home and rest and take some ibuprofen for the pain, and he would discuss the results with me in a few days.

At my next RE visit, the doctor showed me pictures of the hole in my uterus. He told me he didn't understand why it happened, but that my uterus seemed to look okay. This RE somehow missed the fact that my uterus was completely blocked with adhesions. He now suggested that I have a diagnostic laparoscopy to view my internal workings, since the HSG was a failure. Well, my bad luck didn't stop there. During my laparoscopy, the dye to fill my uterus and tubes spilled out through the open puncture wound in my uterus. At my next office visit, the RE discussed with me that I once again had an unsuccessful dye test, but went on to tell me that it seemed as though things looked okay from what he could see during the exam. At the time, I fully believed him, since he was the doctor and I was the patient. After that, I was started on several months of unsuccessful Clomid cycles, and it was no fun. I already suffered from PMS with my periods, and being on Clomid magnified my irritability times 10. At times I think my husband wished he could stay at work all night just to avoid being near me with my horrible mood swings.

After the unsuccessful Clomid cycles, we went on to injectable medications with intrauterine insemination (IUI). The injections were awful

… and remember how I mentioned irritability on Clomid? Well, being on the injectables was even worse than Clomid on my mood. There would be days that I would just start crying in the middle of the day over nothing … literally nothing. I could be sitting on the couch doing a puzzle and the tears would start flowing.

I wasn't able to give myself the needles, and they had to be done at the same time each day, so my husband had to make sure he was home from work in time to give me the shot each night. One night, he wasn't able to come home and I panicked. I ended up having to drive 45 minutes away to my best friend's house so she could give me the shot. And on one occasion when my husband gave me the shot, we don't know what happened, but my skin bubbled up during the shot and it was much more painful than usual. During this time my moods were so unstable, I was completely miserable, and to top it all off, we still weren't getting pregnant. Little did we know at the time that all these medications were worthless because of the adhesions in my uterus!

The next fun part (yeah, right!) was the intrauterine inseminations (IUI). My husband was a trooper through all of this and was willing to participate in whatever he had to do. Luckily we lived only 20 minutes from the RE's office, so my husband was able to produce his "specimen" at home. Our instructions were to wrap the "specimen jar" in a tube sock and put the tube sock under my shirt against my stomach to keep the "specimen" body temperature. Talk about ridiculous! It was quite an adventure, praying that there would be no traffic issues on the way to the doctor's office, as the "specimen" had to arrive within an hour. On top of that, the IUI's were very painful for me. The doctor always had trouble getting the scope into my uterus, and he just shrugged it off and told me he didn't understand why it would be so painful for me.

So, after an unsuccessful year full of mood swings, depression, frustration, and sadness, I started to get a feeling in my gut that something just wasn't right with what we were doing. And let me tell you right now…LISTEN TO YOUR GUT! Don't ignore it! And I'm so glad I listened, because we finally ended up heading in the right direction after I did.

YEAR THREE: THE MIRACLE WORKER

I was really starting to feel like my RE wasn't treating me properly, after having gone through my punctured uterus, the failed laparoscopy, and what I believed to be way too many hormones. At that point, I decided it was time for us to seek a second opinion. My husband and I started asking around, and one day we both came home with a referral to the same doctor … now if that wasn't a sign, I don't know what is!

Right from the start, I immediately knew we were in the right place when this new RE sat down to talk with us. After reviewing my history, he told us that it sounded like I may have intrauterine adhesions. This was the first time I had ever heard of anything like that. How was I able to go an entire year with another RE that never even mentioned that possible reason for my issues? I still don't have an answer to that one. Anyway, my new RE explained to me that if there were adhesions, he could perform surgery to remove them. This all sounded like good news to me and I was ready to get started. Of course, the first test he wanted to perform was an office hysteroscopy and an HSG exam. Oh no, I thought. I don't want another hole in my uterus! I explained my concern to him, and he assured me that he would be very delicate during the procedure and he would stop immediately if he had any issues or if I had any discomfort. I finally felt like I was in good hands with him.

My first procedure with my new RE was an office hysteroscopy. This exam is where the doctor inserts a scope with a camera on the end of it up into your uterus to take a look around. Remembering his promise to be especially gentle with me, he attempted to perform this procedure very slowly and cautiously. I started having some discomfort, so he immediately stopped the exam. Thank you doctor! My HSG was also completed just as he had promised … very delicately … and sure enough, my uterus was a maze of approximately 90% adhesions. I hadn't had any previous surgeries, so, to this day, I have no idea how these adhesions came to be … whether my uterus had always been like that, whether I had a pelvic infection at some point that I never knew about that caused the adhesions, or something else altogether. Nevertheless, we finally had a reason for my infertility, and that alone felt like such a huge weight had been lifted off my shoulders. I honestly felt like half my battle had been won at this point, because not knowing the reason for your infertility can drive a woman insane.

Now that my doctor had visual evidence, via HSG, of my intrauterine adhesions, it was time to set up a laparoscopy to surgically remove them. My surgery went well, and along with the 90% adhesions in my uterus, I also had endometriosis and adhesions along my ascending and descending colon. My doctor was a wonderful surgeon and was able to remove all of the adhesions and endometriosis. I went home from the surgery with a balloon in my uterus with a Foley catheter and a leg bag tied around my leg. It wasn't fun, but it was necessary to help prevent the uterine walls from sticking together again. I was in excruciating pain for several days after my surgery, and because of all the pain medication I was on, I didn't realize that I wasn't able to urinate (I only had little drops coming out, but I assumed it was because I was dehydrated). I ended up in such severe pain that I had to go back to the doctor. He realized I had a distended bladder and emptied it for me! He then sent me home with a second leg bag and another catheter, this one for my bladder. So, for a week I was walking around with two leg bags tied around my legs with tight rubber bands. It was a very long week, needless to say!

At my follow-up office visit, the doctor showed me a video of the actual work he performed on me … it was amazing to see the inside of my uterus and watch the instruments cutting away at all the adhesions! The next plan was to take Premarin for two more weeks and then Provera for a withdrawal bleed. Surprisingly, I had what I would consider a "normal" period that month … I actually had to wear a regular size pad for two days because I actually had some flow (I typically only needed to use a panty liner)! And on top of that, my bowel movements were better too due to the fact that he removed the adhesions from my colon (I know, too much information, right!).

During my next office visit, I received wonderful news from my doctor. He performed an office hysteroscopy … and remember the last time when I was in terrible discomfort and he had to stop the procedure? Well, this time was completely different! It didn't hurt at all, and he was able to easily insert the scope with the camera into my uterus to find a "totally normal cavity with no evidence of any adhesions present." What an incredible surgeon! Our next step, since I had long cycles, was to try a few cycles with Clomid with an hCG trigger injection and IUI. I decided I would try one month with the drugs, but after that we were going to try naturally. Well, that cycle was a bust, so we decided to start trying on our own.

At this point I had started taking my basal body temperature, charting, and using ovulation kits each month. I was so determined to get pregnant that I would literally lie in bed for a half an hour after sex with a pillow under my butt for gravity to help things along! After four months of natural cycles, a miracle happened...I got a positive pregnancy test! I was shaking so much from excitement, I could hardly believe it! We immediately told our family, and my dad left the nicest congratulations message on my answering machine that I listened to it every day for weeks!

YEAR FOUR: STARTING OVER AGAIN

Unfortunately, things went really wrong once again. At our 12-week-ultrasound, the baby had no heartbeat, when just a few weeks prior the baby had been fine. At this point, I had been seeing my regular OB/GYN, who determined I had a "missed abortion," and told me a D&C would be my best option. It was the night before I was going to tell everyone at my work that I was pregnant. When I think back to that day, even now, I can still feel the deep, deep heartbreak and sorrow when the doctor broke the news to me. I was stunned. I couldn't stop crying. I had to ask my husband to make all the phone calls to our family, because I just couldn't say the words out loud. My heart ached so badly. One of the worst things of all was that I had to wait four impossibly long days before I could go in for a D&C I stayed in bed. I didn't want to get up. I didn't want to do anything but cry and grieve. When I called my boss to tell him I would be out for the week, he broke some other bad news to me. Apparently, a coworker of mine was also about to tell everyone that she was three months pregnant, and she had an ultrasound on the same day as me and received the same terrible news. When I came back to work the following week, we talked and cried, and talked and cried. Work was different after that. In fact, everything was different after that. My life had changed forever.

I started a journal, and one of my first entries said, "I'm so depressed and I feel so inadequate ... I don't think I've ever struggled with anything so hard in my life ... I don't feel like myself anymore ... I feel lost ... I feel like a stranger in my own skin… I want my old self back … I want to be pregnant again … desperately." My miscarriage had devastated me. It had hardened me to the world, and I knew that I'd no longer be able to have an innocent, care-free pregnancy. The miscarriage robbed me of that. I knew that if I ever got pregnant again, I'd be trapped in fear of worrying that this would happen again.

Thankfully, I found an extremely supportive website about trying to conceive after miscarriage, and I spent hours and hours each day on the site. I made many "virtual friends" through the site, and I was able to share my story about my Asherman's and my successful treatment. The website became an obsession for me, but it was what I needed at the time.

At this point, I was now officially obsessed with trying to get pregnant. It was the only thing in the world that I wanted. Three months after my D&C, I had some bleeding in my luteal phase … to the point that I had to run home from work and change my pants! I was hoping that it was due to implantation, because the timing was right. Unfortunately, my period came, and I decided it was time to go and see my RE again, and yes, I received even more bad news. At this point I was really beginning to wonder how much bad news one person could take. My RE performed an operative hysteroscopy on me, and it turned out that during my D&C, the doctor who performed it didn't remove all of the "products of conception," which is why I had that strange bleeding in my luteal phase three months later. I was horrified.

You see, when I went in for my D&C, my normal gynecologist was unavailable, so I had to have a doctor I had never seen before. I had explained to him that I had a history of Asherman's, that I had seen an RE, and I was concerned about the Asherman's coming back after the D&C. He told me he would be extra cautious and he would perform everything manually. Well, apparently, he didn't do a very good job. I immediately changed my gynecologist after that, as I never wanted to see that doctor's face again.

So, now we were back to square one, and I was desperately sad. At this point, my friends and family were starting to ask hard questions like "When is it enough? At what point do you decide you're not meant to have children?" I know my family and friends were saying these things out of concern, but to me, it felt like a knife in my back. I wanted a child and I wasn't going to stop, at least not yet. I wasn't ready to give up yet. At this point I had gotten pregnant once, so I felt like I could get pregnant again.

After my operative hysteroscopy, my RE once again inserted a balloon catheter in my uterus to make sure I didn't form any new adhesions. I was also put on Premarin and Provera again. At this point, due to my extreme sadness from the miscarriage, I knew it was time to see a therapist. My RE referred me to a wonderful therapist who specialized in infertility, and she was able to help me deal with my grief.

Just when I thought I was dealing with a clean slate and was able to start trying to conceive again, the bad news continued to come … my adhesions had returned! For several months, I didn't bleed at all from my period, so my RE performed another office hysteroscopy and was unable to even get the scope through my cervix into my uterus. Apparently, a new band of adhesions had formed at the bottom of my uterus. The RE tried several attempts to break through the adhesions with the scope, but was unsuccessful. The following week my RE was on vacation, and I was seen by the other doctor in the practice. He also tried to perform an office hysteroscopy, but with no success. The following week I went back for a third office hysteroscopy, and this time the RE used an extremely small instrument and was able to actually get through the band of adhesions and into my uterus. He decided we should perform another HSG to see how the rest of my uterus and tubes looked. It did appear that I still had a few small adhesions toward the bottom of my uterus, but everything else looked good. He didn't believe that those adhesions would preclude me from getting pregnant and the band that had been blocking my cervix was successfully broken apart during my last office hysteroscopy.

YEAR FIVE: 100 PREGNANCY TESTS

Now that I had been given clearance to start trying to conceive again, I was going all out. I was still madly obsessed with my message boards and I was charting my temperature daily without missing a day. I had even gone online and purchased a bundle of 100 pregnancy tests through E-bay. Yes, you read that correctly … 100 pregnancy tests. During my luteal phase, I would start using pregnancy tests seven days after ovulation. Oh, and during the cycles when I used the hCG trigger injection, the injection would give you an immediate false positive result; so, I would take a pregnancy test every day in the beginning of my luteal phase until it became negative 7 to 10 days later, and that way I would know that if I got a positive test after that, it would be the real thing. I did mention that I was obsessed, right?

At this point my doctor recommended that I do a natural cycle with monitoring. That meant no medications, but I would go in for the ultrasound monitoring of my follicle growth. This was a particularly long cycle for me, and it seemed like I was never going to ovulate. My follicles just weren't growing during this cycle, and my RE recommended we stop trying, and on the next cycle we would start Femara, because Clomid was giving me a thin endometrial lining. I wasn't sure I liked the idea of using Femara, as it was primarily used as a breast cancer drug, but at this point I was willing to do anything that my RE asked me to do … well, almost anything. My RE told us not to have unprotected sex that month, because it seemed like I had a "bad egg." He explained that this meant that the egg was growing so slowly, and if I did get pregnant, it would up my chances of having a miscarriage. He told me he would give me Provera to bring on my period so we could start with the Femara as soon as my next cycle began. I was distraught at the fact that we'd have to skip a cycle at this point. I kept going back and forth with my friends on my message board about what I should do. They were all in the same boat as me … they didn't know if it was better for me to listen to my doctor's advice, or just go ahead and try to conceive anyway … not like I had much chance of getting pregnant, with my past history!

It just so happened that my husband and I had a trip to Disney World planned during this time. On our trip, I took the Provera like my doctor had prescribed, but we decided to have sex anyway. I brought along some ovulation tests, but they were all negative anyway. I tried really hard to enjoy our trip, but the entire time I just kept thinking about trying to get pregnant. I was trying to time everything in my head about when my period would come and how soon we could begin trying again.

When we got home from our Disney trip, my 100 pregnancy tests had arrived in the mail (which I proceeded to immediately hide from my husband, because he really didn't need to know I was *that* obsessed!) I decided I would try one out, just to make sure they actually worked. You see, it was only $20.00 for the entire lot, and normally they are $20.00 for one when you buy them at the store! But these were the cheap kind … tiny little strips, where you have to pee in a cup, and then dip the strip in the urine and wait. Well, when I tried the first one, I followed all the instructions, and the stupid strip showed up positive! I couldn't believe that I had just wasted $20.00 on a batch of faulty pregnancy tests! My initial reaction was that I was so mad, but deep down inside I started questioning myself as to how this would be possible.

The next morning was bittersweet. It was Thanksgiving Day, and my parents, with whom I am very close and have always lived very close to me, were moving to Florida from our hometown of Philadelphia, and they were driving down that day to start their new retired life. My mother has lung problems and was able to breathe better in the cleaner Florida air. They had been living with us for about two months after they sold their house up here and were waiting for their house in Florida to be completed. After I sadly gave them their good-bye hugs and saw them out the door, I decided to try another one of those faulty pregnancy tests. I thought, "Could they all be faulty?" Sure enough, once again it showed up positive. I proceeded to dip another eight tests into the urine cup, and sure enough, all of them were positive. I couldn't believe this was happening, so I immediately went out to the store to buy two of the $20.00-for-one pregnancy tests. I always have to pee a lot, so I didn't have a problem having to go right away when I got home again. And guess what – this time, the test had words on it, and it said "PREGNANT!!!" I was stunned. I didn't know what to say or do. I was shaking and trembling like there was an earthquake inside of me. I started pacing around the room like a caged tiger. I was astounded. After calming down, I picked up the phone and called my husband to tell him the crazy/wonderful/unbelievable news. He was in disbelief. I think he asked, "How?" I didn't have an answer for him. And to make me crazier, it was Thanksgiving Day, so my doctor's office was closed and I wasn't able to call them to get any blood work done! That was the longest Thanksgiving Day of my entire life!

The following day I called my doctor and they had me come in right away. Shockingly, my blood work proved that I was a few days pregnant.

The nurses and my RE were stunned. One of the nurses said to me, "How did this happen?" Apparently, after looking back on my temperature chart, the Provera that I took to bring on my withdrawal bleed ending up causing me to ovulate instead (which can happen in rare cases). We actually had sex a full five days before I ovulated … just about the longest amount of time that sperm can survive before meeting up with an egg.

As the weeks went on, my blood work continued to rise, and the ultrasounds started showing the makings of our baby. During one appointment, my RE exclaimed, "I'm good, aren't I!" and "How 'bout that uterus!" I was so nervous as the weeks went on, especially as it got closer to the 12-week-mark, which is about the time that we had our previous miscarriage. During one of my appointments, my RE checked my heartbeat and noted it to be 108 beats per minute! My doctor told me I really needed to start controlling my anxiety. I tried my best, but that's easier said than done. After about 10 weeks of a good-looking, healthily progressing pregnancy, it was time for me to say good-bye to my RE and move on to my new gynecologist. It was such a bittersweet moment, as my RE had been through so much with me. I couldn't explain to him in words how grateful I was to him for everything he had done for me … from removing all of my adhesions (more than once!) to just being so kind, understanding, and gentle with me. We said our good-byes and I was off to start seeing my regular gynecologist. This was a new gynecologist that I had never seen before, and he's actually wonderful as well. He had an ultrasound machine right in his office, so I was able to get many ultrasounds through my pregnancy.

Of course I didn't have the easiest of pregnancies. I bled a full two weeks in the first trimester, I had very bad morning sickness, I had early contractions and was put on bed rest, I fell and dislocated my sacroiliac joint and had to be put on pain medicine, and the baby was breech so I had to have a C-section, and I ended up with severe postpartum depression, but overall, it was all worth it. Why, you ask? Well, remember that "bad egg" my RE had told me about? Well, that bad egg is now my beautiful, healthy, happy three-and-a-half year old daughter, and she was worth every bit of our struggle!

Now, almost four years later, my husband and I have decided not to try to conceive any more children. Because of all the mental and physical anguish that having Asherman's has caused me, I know in my heart of hearts that I couldn't bare to go through it all again. I still have painful periods with practically no flow, and I've recently gotten a tubal ligation. Coming to this decision was very difficult. My husband and I talk on and off about the idea of adoption. Sometimes we're very saddened that our little girl will be an only child, especially when she asks us if she can have a sibling to play with her. Ultimately, I know this is the best decision for my family and me, as I know I would not have the strength to try to conceive again. To this day, and forever, my life will be changed, and I pray that the awareness of Asherman's grows to the point that every patient is informed and treated properly in their care of intrauterine adhesions.

III. ADOPTION

23. THERESA

My husband and I were married in July 2001. I was 35 years old and we both knew that we couldn't wait too long to start having children. We were trained in the highly scientific method of natural family planning. And it worked like a charm. We started trying to get pregnant in September of 2002, and conceived the very next month. We were ecstatic! For some reason I always thought that I would be one of those people who would have a problem getting pregnant.

But here I was, due to have a baby in July 2003. Before I was even married, I always thought that the best time to have a baby was in the summer. I fantasized about having really fun birthday parties outside with a moon bounce and pony rides, water ice and three-legged races. It's just something I always thought about. It's the reason why we started trying to get pregnant when we did.

We decided to tell our family about our news on Christmas Eve. We couldn't wait. In the meantime, we had an ultrasound and saw our baby's heartbeat at 7.5 weeks. It was amazing! Christmas Eve day came along and I just didn't feel right. Part of me thought that I was just really nervous about telling everyone the news later on that day. I don't really like being the center of attention. But part of me thought that there was something wrong with the baby. So I called my doctor's office and gave them my vague symptoms of not feeling right. Since it was Christmas Eve, I could tell they really didn't want to add another patient to the list, but with some coaxing, they agreed. And then our world was shattered when they couldn't find the heartbeat.

I then had to make the terrible decision as to how the miscarriage should proceed. Because I was afraid that the miscarriage might happen while I was at work, I opted for surgical intervention. And this is where all of my problems started. I remember waking up in the recovery room. The surgeon came to speak to me and told me that my uterus was retro-verted, which means it tilts back. He told me that he had had a hard time reaching the fetus and that he had to scrape a lot.

Little did I know that this was only the very beginning of a crazy ride on a very emotional rollercoaster. I'm not much of a rider on the physical rollercoaster, but the emotional ones are even scarier.

In September of 2003, we decided to start trying to conceive again. So with our handy and accurate natural family planning charting, and lots of conversations with God, we began all over again, assuming we would be able to conceive as quickly as the first time. But seven months went by and nothing happened. At this point, I also noticed that my periods changed from lasting five days to about two days with much less bleeding.

We decided it was time to see a reproductive endocrinologist in our area. At my first appointment, the doctor attempted to do an HSG (hysterosalpinogram) but the scope was unable to pass through my cervix. He told me to come back the next day and he would try again. This time, he stuck what looked like a huge needle and tried to "poke" through my cervix.

I've never felt so much pain. Tears just rolled down my face. Still unable to pass anything through my cervix, he told me we needed to talk about my options.

At this point, I didn't have much trust in this doctor so, I decided to do some research on my own. This was when I stumbled upon the Asherman´s website. I wrote in my symptoms to Poly, the moderator of the group, and she diagnosed me with Asherman´s Syndrome.

My husband and I picked one of the A-list doctor from the Asherman´s site and drove a few hundred miles for our appointment. We felt confident right away after our meeting with this doctor that he knew what he was doing. He had state of the art equipment in his office and performed a sonohystogram and was able to see that I had complete scarring of my entire cervical canal.

This would explain why the previous doctor couldn't get anything through and why my period was so light. But my A-list doctor was able to dilate my cervix in the office to 2 cm. However, I had much more going on. I still needed surgical intervention.

And all of this was because of the doctor who took it upon himself to scrape my uterus to smithereens. How I wish I had chosen to let the miscarriage happen on its own! So I went on to have surgery. My operative report stated that I had severe adhesions and severe endometriosis in different areas of my uterus. I also still needed my cervix dilated. Everything went well during surgery. I continued to see this A-list doctor for all my follow-up appointments. A few months later, I needed my cervix dilated again and he was able to do this conveniently in his office.

With the surgery over with, Joe and I decided to see another reproductive endocrinologist in our area. Our A-list doctor knew of him and said that he was pretty aggressive. We were happy to hear this because that's who we needed! We started seeing this new doctor and we explained to him that we were Catholic and we wanted very much to follow the Catholic doctrine which means that we didn't want any kind of reproductive therapy that went against the Catholic Church. If we couldn't conceive a baby without having intercourse, then we didn't want that treatment. This doctor totally followed our wishes and worked with us. According to the Catholic Church we were allowed to use medications to assist us to conceive while having intercourse.

From October 2005 to July 2006 I was put on several different medications. I also had 23 acupuncture treatments to try to lower my FSH (follicle stimulating hormone) level. We decided to stop treatment when we were picking up another dose of the medication and the pharmacist pulled us aside to tell us that after this dose our insurance will run out. We had reached the $15,000 coverage allotted for fertility medications. If we were to pay for this specific medication out of pocket, it would have cost us $2,600!!

This is when we knew that God had other plans for us. Joe and I had talked about adoption even before we were married. It was something that always intrigued me. We also have two nieces that were adopted, so it didn't seem too out of the ordinary to pursue. We prayed a lot about it and decided we wanted to go with an adoption agency that was small.

The one we chose was perfect for us. There was a lot of paperwork to get through and lots of regulations to cover but we had all of our paperwork in by March 2007. At this time, I was really comfortable with the fact that we were going to be parents to a baby that was not biologically ours. We were both emotionally ready and in the end it didn't really matter to us how we became parents. I was 41 years old at this point and I actually couldn't even imagine being pregnant.

Seven months later, in October 2007, my period was late by one week. I took a pregnancy test and it was positive!!! We were shocked! We weren't trying, charting or praying for this to happen. Again, we were able to see the baby's heartbeat, but again it ended in miscarriage. This time I opted to let it happen on its own and we started back with the adoption plan.

In June of 2008 we were chosen by a birthmother to be the parents to her unborn baby who was due to be born in August 2008. We went out to meet the birthparents in July but didn't really feel secure that the adoption was going to go through. We didn't really connect with them. It didn't feel right. We weren't shocked when they changed their minds the day their baby was born. There were so many issues with them that we were actually fine that it didn't work out.

We felt that there had to be a better situation out there for us. Then two months later, on October 12, 2008, we were chosen by another set of birth parents whose baby girl was due in nine days! We went out to meet them three days after they chose us, and we all got along so well! It just felt right. It felt like we had known them our entire lives and they said the same of us. The birthmother wanted me to be in the delivery room, so I had the privilege of seeing my daughter being born and being able to cut her umbilical cord.

Our daughter, Serena Ann, is now 16 months old and we can't imagine life without her. We talk about how we wish we never even wasted time with the fertility drugs. We wish we went straight to adoption. But we also realize that you must take steps to be able to get to the adoption option. You must be emotionally ready and sometimes you have to go through many painful steps to get there.

We also believe that God makes things happen for a reason. If we had not gone through the fertility drugs and had that other adoption not fallen through, we would not have our Serena with us. We would have had a different baby. Joe and I honestly believe that God knew we were to be her parents before she was even born.

The most amazing thing is that we forget that she is not our biological child. I have a few embarrassing stories where I told my pediatrician that I was afraid Serena was going to inherit some issues of mine like my acne as a child and the fact that I'm allergic to a lot of different kinds of fruit. And the doctor looked at me funny both times and reminded me, "She's adopted, right?" And I say, "Oh yeah, I keep forgetting that!"

24. DARLENE

My husband and I had always considered adoption. We were together for seven years before marrying, and as soon as we decided that we wanted children, our first thought was to adopt. My husband's uncle, whom he is very close to, was adopted. Many of my friends in childhood were adopted. Why have a baby biologically when there are so many children who need parents? However, it seemed "easier", and potentially more fun, to conceive a child and give birth. From the start, however, I decided that I would rather adopt rather than jeopardize my health and finances pursuing extensive fertility treatment, if it came to that.

So, I stopped taking birth control, went for a preconception physical, and we started trying to conceive a child. I never menstruated regularly, and even called it my "biannual event" when I was in college. My gynecologist had said that if we didn't conceive within six months, we should return for a follow-up appointment. However, after not menstruating for four months, I called my doctor, who thought I probably wasn't ovulating, and recommended Clomid. Clomid sounded relatively benign, and it seemed pretty similar to taking the pill which I had taken for years, so I decided to try it. After the fact I realized it could have some significant side effects which luckily I did not experience.

Once on the Clomid and taking my temperature to tell if I was ovulating, within a few months I was pregnant. We were so excited! We told the world. At my 8 week ultrasound, the fetus looked smaller than would be expected and by the end of the first trimester, I miscarried. I went in for a confirmatory ultrasound the day I started bleeding and the fetus had been absorbed by my body. I was given the usual options to rid myself of the remaining "products of conception": Wait and let it all happen on its own, try drug therapy to bring on miscarriage, or D&C. I immediately chose D&C. I don't remember the risks of the different options being discussed, not that they weren't … I just don't remember. I know "Asherman's" was never specifically discussed. However, it wouldn't have mattered if it had. All I wanted was for "it" to be over … NOW, so I could move on and get pregnant again. Also, in retrospect, given what I now know about my body, I would have ended up with a D&C anyway. No regrets on that front. I had the D&C that day.

My hormone levels took longer than expected to come down to normal. After a few months, I went on Clomid again. Shortly afterwards, I had a strange bleeding episode which didn't look like menstruation. An ultrasound showed nothing but a highly stimulated ovary from the Clomid. Everything else seemed normal. I menstruated and ovulated as expected. We tried to conceive for a few months without success.

At that point my gynecologist referred us to a fertility specialist. I am not sure why we didn't just try to adopt instead of trying more fertility treatments. The fertility treatments we tried to that point seemed benign and had been effective. Trying to conceive still felt "easier" than adopting. We went for a consultation to see what was recommended. They did some tests on my husband, and his sperm seemed healthy. The fertility specialist recommended that we try inseminations to increase our likelihood of conceiving.

We tried a few unsuccessful inseminations. Then I was sent for a hysterosalpingogram (HSG). As soon as they injected the dye into my uterus, I felt immense pain. I could see on the monitor that the dye was going nowhere. That was when I found out my uterus was blocked at the cervix, though there was no way to tell the extent of the blockage.

I had never heard of Asherman's. The radiologist didn't mention Asherman's by name. The nurse who called me with the results of the HSG didn't say "Asherman's". She actually told me my fallopian tubes were blocked. Luckily, I had a copy of the radiology report and knew enough from my background to know that "fallopian tubes not visualized" did not mean my fallopian tubes were blocked, it just meant that the radiologist never visualized them. When I finally met with my fertility specialist, Asherman's Syndrome was first described to me. I was told that surgery via laparoscopy and hysteroscopy was the best option, but that they wouldn't know if my case was correctable until they were actually in my uterus, since they couldn't determine the extent of the scarring.

I went home and googled Asherman's. One of the first listings that came up was the ashermans.org website. I immediately joined the email group. The information available through the website was far more extensive than any other resource I could find.

I don't know if I would have had the surgery if its purpose was solely to restore fertility. However, the other health complications of Asherman's and my insurance company's coverage of it made the decision easy. My fertility specialist happened to be the only surgeon in the state who performs the procedure, though at the time I didn't fully explore the ashermans.org surgeon list. The procedure lasted several hours and I was told that the scarring was quite severe, completely filling my uterus and the worst the surgeon ever managed to successfully correct. An IUD (Intrauterine Device) was placed in my uterus to hold it open and I was treated with estrogen therapy for a few months before the IUD was removed.

We decided to try again. Knowing that it might not be possible for me to get pregnant, we also started looking into adoption alternatives at the same time. After a few unsuccessful inseminations, I was sent for another

HSG. It showed some recurrent scarring over my cervix. The radiologist proceeded with the scan to break up the scarring and I conceived that month for the second time.

The weekend after I found out that I was pregnant, my husband and I attended an annual adoption conference hosted by a local adoption support group. At that point, we were considering both international and domestic adoption. The afternoon of the conference was dedicated to comparing and contrasting on every level the various types of adoption. We left the conference both favoring local domestic open adoption of a newborn. Open adoption means that all of the participants in the adoption know one another, though the degree to which there is contact between the adoptive and birth family varies. Usually in an open adoption the birth mother chooses the adoptive family. Though historically not the norm, currently adoption advocates in the United States favor open adoption and it is believed to be the most psychologically healthy form of adoption for all parties involved. Having a relationship with our child's birth family appealed to my husband and me. We felt it would benefit our child, and might mitigate some of the loss experienced by the birth family. Also, adopting in the United States seemed like the right thing to do for us, especially once we understood the laws of Oregon governing adoption which were a little less onerous for adoptive parents than some states. And we wanted the opportunity to adopt a newborn, which would be difficult internationally.

Later that month, there was no fetal heartbeat detected on the 5-week-ultrasound when there should have been a heartbeat. I was sent for a confirmatory high resolution ultrasound which showed that the fetus was not viable. Although devastated, I had reached the end of pursuing fertility treatment. For us, conceiving a baby was not easy. It had been three years of pain, uncertainty, and expense. All this with no promise of a baby in sight was too high of a price to pay just to have our baby come out of my body. There were babies coming out of other people's bodies that were as amazing as any my husband and I could produce. I went through the house and dumped anything related to fertility, books, medications, thermometers, graphs, into the kitchen trash (a bit of a surprise to my husband when he threw something away later that day). I looked at all of the websites of the local adoption agencies. Due to our spiritual and political leanings, there was only one agency that fit. That agency also placed the largest number of infants in our state, all in open adoptions. I scheduled us for an information session the next month.

This time around, a D&C was not an option due to the Asherman's. I took several rounds of various medications before, four months later, I miscarried. By then, we had taken our required adoption class and were working on our home study and paperwork. The paperwork for the adoption was onerous. In addition to questionnaires, fingerprints, photo collages and official copies of documents, there were personal accounts and letters to write as part of the process. My husband struggled with the autobiography, while I found the "Dear Birthmother" letter the biggest challenge. It took rocking in a rocking chair while knitting to calm me down enough to work on it with my husband. Finalizing the paperwork consumed six months. Though difficult, it was easier than the uncertainty of conceiving, since there was definitely a baby at the end of the process.

We entered the adoptive parent pool and six months later we adopted our son. It was an eventful time. I occupied the wait knitting baby clothes and wishing for the phone to ring. It felt like a popularity contest - someone needed to like you best, but your whole future depended upon it. Then there was the "disruption". After waiting in the pool for four and a half months, we were selected by a birth family, but the birth mother changed her mind about putting her son up for adoption while in labor. As painful as the waiting was, as the cliché goes, it was all worth it.

My husband and I joke that we went to dinner and came back with a baby. Though an exaggeration, it is not that far from the truth. About six weeks after our previous disappointment, we received a call that there was a birth mother due in two weeks who wanted to meet us. We drove a few hours away to meet her and her family, including grandfather, aunts and uncle, with the agency social worker, for dinner. The family had all read our profile and they had definitely decided we were "mom and dad." We got to know them, but they already knew us. It was a strange feeling. Their conviction and confidence were infectious. They asked us to spend the night and meet them the next day for the second mediation which is the next step in the process. We found a hotel and met the social worker the next day in the cafeteria where our son's birthmother was having a prenatal exam. The social worker received a call while we were waiting. Our son's birthmother had preeclampsia and was being admitted for labor to be induced immediately.

We had the second meditation in a birthing suite and everything went smoothly, from finalizing the birth plan, to deciding on details together such as whether to circumcise our son and whether we would like to hold an entrustment ceremony at some point after the birth. Every member of the birth family loved the name that we tentatively chose for our son and it quickly became more than tentative, as they started referring to him with that name from that point forward. At around 6 am the next morning, our son was delivered by Cesarean section and wheeled in to meet us. I vaguely remember someone in our son's birth family pushing us forward and introducing us to our son.

We spent four days in the hospital together. My husband stayed in a pediatric room nearby which the hospital made available to us. Our son's birth mother asked me to stay in her room with her and our son. She was young, still very sick, and scared to be in the hospital. I took care of both her and Joshua each night until our tearful entrustment ceremony on the morning our son was three days old. I have never been more sad, elated, and exhausted all at the same time, and it was perfect. I cannot imagine the depths of the loss felt by our son's birth mother, but, as I have had the fortune to be able to tell her, I will be forever grateful for her selfless courage and for choosing us as our son's parents.

There is life, love, and happiness despite and because of Asherman's.

IV. MOVING ON

25. LOUISE

Unknown to me at the time, my Asherman's story, and biggest grief, began the exact same time my son, and greatest joy, was born. My severe Asherman's came about by a birth injury in relation to an emergency C-section on August 17th, 2004. After two and a half years, I was finally diagnosed on February 21st, 2007. I had never before had any kind of uterine surgery, D&C or prior pregnancy which could have caused my Asherman's. As a maternity patient carrying my first child, I was admitted to an emergency C-section for severe fetal distress (very low heartbeat detectable) in the very late hours of August 16th, 2004, after 6-8 hours of labor. My son was delivered healthy by an experienced consultant at a private birth unit in North West London, UK, on August 17th, 2004. I seemingly recovered quickly and suffered only minor problems with the suture not dissolving as they should. The sutures were removed manually a few weeks later.

The day after the birth a midwife kindly suggested that I consult a cranial osteopath to check my baby and myself, as the birth had been long and quite tough on us both. I agreed to have a session, which concluded we were both fine. It would have been more beneficial to offer a consultation on the events leading to the emergency C-section, including the potential complications and risks of the surgery. I was never presented with the content of the consent form and was not made aware of the most common as well rare complications of an emergency C-section. I have since obtained my medical records from the birth unit and noticed that the particular consent form does not list any complications. There did not seem to be any procedure in place at the birth unit to discuss complications and risks with the patient after an emergency C-section.

At my six-week-checkup, my obstetrician advised that a vaginal examination was not necessary since I did not give birth naturally. She told me the reason being, that nothing had changed down there! She did not mention that something could have changed IN there! I was never worried, as I believed and trusted to be in safe hands in the care of a consultant affiliated with a world- renowned birth unit, which claims to offer excellent and outstanding care.

I wanted to and was encouraged to breastfeed my baby and did so for nearly five months and awaited my first period. My periods were more painful than I recall them being before the birth of my son, as well as shorter and lighter. I did not think much of it at the time. I had a routine examination with my regular obstetrician a few months later and he concluded that the results were normal. In the early summer of 2006 my husband and I actively started trying to conceive a second child, but did not succeed. As our first child was conceived very easily (first attempt) as well as having the now irregular (ranging from 23-30 days) lighter and more painful periods, I booked an appointment with my obstetrician for another checkup in November 2006. The doctor requested a vaginal ultrasound, which indicated a small area of white lesions in the uterine cavity (fundus). I was told it could be a tiny (perhaps calcified submucous) fibroid. I remember referring to and specifically asking if my problems conceiving could have anything to do with my C-section, which my obstetrician did not confirm nor elaborate on any further.

A few weeks later I received a letter from my obstetrician recommending me to see a fertility expert, because the possibility of a very small fibroid in the uterine cavity could prevent further pregnancy. I consulted the fertility doctor on January 2nd, 2007. The doctor performed an ultrasound, which indicated that my uterine cavity was divided by possibly intrauterine adhesions or an intrauterine fibroid. When I asked him if my condition could be caused by having had a C-section, he also declined with the explanation that a C-section scar is located lower in the uterus. He did not mention that injury could occur when manually removing the placenta or otherwise in relation to a C-section surgery. The doctor suggested performing a hysteroscopy/laparoscopy to divide/remove the adhesions and/or fibroids with a laser. When I asked about risks of this kind of surgery, the doctor did not elaborate. My husband and I did not feel confident to pursue any treatment in his care.

We decided to get a second opinion and consulted another obstetrician on February 21st, 2007. The doctor performed a 3-D ultrasound and clearly diagnosed me with severe intrauterine adhesions and a thin and deficient C-section scar. He recommended a hysteroscopy to remove the adhesions and to choose a surgeon with expertise in this kind of delicate surgery.

At this point I had become a member of the Asherman's site and had received help and support about the condition, that I so wished I did not have. I remember after my diagnosis returning to the site informing the members that I have Asherman's, feeling a part of something warm and welcoming. From the site I had learned that I should choose a good and experienced surgeon in order to avoid acquiring additional scarring. I also know now, that any surgery will leave scarring and that surgery most often needs to be repeated several times in order to correct the issue. I had read a lot of encouraging stories on the site of women conceiving naturally thereafter and following an almost normal pregnancy and normal natural birth. However, I also listened and heard stories from women who had to struggle and suffer quite traumatically in an attempt to get pregnant. Many of these women had premature births and post natal consequences which was a real and scary fact for me to consider.

We decided I should go for surgery in March 2007 to remove the adhesions inside my uterus. I had pain every month and wanted at least to give it try. I did not know the full extent of the severity of my Asherman's and hoped that I would be one of those women who only suffered a mild case. I was puzzled as to how I could have Asherman's since I never had had any D&C or any other kind of uterine disease or infection. I was very anxious and very nervous to have the surgery. Looking back, I did not have any reasons to be so nervous. But, in that period of my life, I was scared and thought all would go wrong with me … wasn't I the one out of a million who got Asherman's from a C-section?

I had an operative hysteroscopy in London by one of the UK´s leading Asherman's surgeons. The surgery went well and, physically, was not a big deal at all. I was at this point emotionally drained from having my whole world turned upside down. The only thing I thought about and cared about was Asherman's and without the web support group I do not think I would have coped as well as I did. My husband was a big support. My family, however, did not really understand and in this period I chatted on the Asherman's support group every day.

At my pre- op consultation, my doctor and surgeon knew immediately of my condition when hearing of my symptoms and clinical history of a C-section. He attempted and successfully removed scar tissue obliterating 77% of my uterine cavity. I had a severe case of intrauterine adhesions. A follow-up hysterosalpingo-gram (HSG) performed in May 2007 showed no reformation of scarring but was inconclusive to whether my tubes were obstructed (corneal occlusion) or if the tubes appeared closed due to tubal spasm.

I have since done a lot of research into intrauterine adhesions/Asherman's Syndrome and mostly received information from members of the Asherman's support group. From my research, Asherman's seems to be a likely diagnosis if a woman has had uterine surgery and complaints of lighter, shorter and irregular periods, possible pain, a history of infertility or (miscarriages) as well as some irregularities on an ultrasound. As adhesions formed within weeks of surgery, I am convinced that the follow-up care I received was not excellent, if even up to standard. I should have been informed of the risks, given a clinical debriefing and information to enable me to take and pursue informed decisions on my after care at the six week checkup. The only thing advice given by my doctor was to wait a year after the C-section before getting pregnant again in order for the scar to heal properly.

After the initial hysteroscopy I recovered over the summer and was so happy just to be pain free. I was struggling emotionally with the pain of it all though, but tried to put the next decision in front of me.

I then went for a follow-up 3D scan in late 2007, which showed that I had approximately 10-25% scarring remaining. I would most likely need another surgery if I was to conceive and to improve chances of a successful pregnancy and birth. I was also informed that although my case improved from severe to moderate/mild, I also had a very thin and deficient C-section scar, which added to my risk profile. There was an increased chance of the egg implanting in the scar with consequences similar to those of an ectopic pregnancy. In any case, I would need a planned C-section in a subsequent birth. My uterus would not bear any contractions in a natural birth.

I was very sad at this point. I felt I might have been able to deal with the Asherman's by now, but my age (37 at the point) and the fact that I also had the C-section scar in my uterus to be concerned about scared me a lot. I managed to book a second hysteroscopy in February 2008, which I later cancelled because I was too scared to face the step after. I went to seek a second opinion in spring 2008 by the second UK recommended Asherman's expert. Upon yet another 3D scan, his opinion was that I would be okay in pursuing another pregnancy. He also recommended a second surgery to remove some of the remaining scarring and to check whether my tubes were in fact open or not. He said that my main problem would probably be getting pregnant and that a second surgery would improve my chances of this happening naturally as opposed to IVF. I was scheduled for surgery in early summer 2008.

Since the summer of 2007 I had not been in a good place about all of this. I envied all the other mothers having a second child at my son's school. I met women who never had a child of their own and felt ashamed for grieving the loss of not having number two. I struggled to cope with the fact that I was not enjoying life as I was before and that the last year of my son's life (from 3-4 years) had been a blur and filled with anxiety. I was lost and sad that my relationship with my husband suffered. Sad I could not give him another child and much more.

Then, one day, approximately two weeks before the date of my planned second surgery, I felt very burdened by it all, so much so, that after a long conversation with my best friend, suddenly realized that I, despite the privilege of having all the support in the world, the best doctor and more, could not pursue the surgery nor a second pregnancy. The unknowns, the time, the effort and the costs in all aspects were too big for me and my husband and my son. My husband and I had had endless talks about emotions and what ifs and so on. We had also talked about acceptance. I was adamant that this should not be an obsession that would make me bitter and lose out any longer of living a "normal" life. I chose to look at my life as it was and found that it was a good life in fact. One that made me happy. I felt grateful for what I had already despite Asherman's and suddenly felt an inner peace in letting go and giving up. I remember thinking that had this ordeal been the fight for getting a first child I would probably have continued the fight … would I have been ten years younger I probably would have fought on … would I not have a thin and deficient C-section scar to deal with on top of having Asherman's, I probably would have opted to fight and have another surgery. But that morning after crying and grieving for hours, I decided that the road to recovery, trying to conceive, conception, carrying a child for nine high risk months, and the birth and possible post-natal consequences on my body would be too much for me. I looked myself in the mirror and decided I had to move on and take on my life again … some would say I gave up. I choose to say, I accepted and embraced life in that moment. And that is what I did. I cancelled the surgery and I never looked back. A burden was lifted from my shoulders. I still feel the relief, but I also know I will always grieve. The people who told me that I did not want "it" enough are wrong. I went through a process and dealt with it with acceptance instead of obsession, because that was the alternative for me. I admire my fellow Asherman's sisters who fight and fought and then gave up or succeeded. But I chose to give up without much of a fight and believe that this was not the easiest decision either. I knew what I had, one son, one husband and a life I love. I was not willing to risk that for the unknown. I hope my story can encourage others to either take the fight, follow their heart or just let go if that is the right decision for them, as it was for me. I do still consider myself a brave woman, a loving mother and a loving wife.

As an end note, I remember the anger and grief I felt about not being informed, debriefed, advised, warned and maybe even diagnosed in a procedure of follow-up care following an emergency C-section. I also wonder if my C-section was performed with care of avoiding adhesions. I therefore asked the birth unit to investigate and provide me with an explanation as to what policies the birth unit had when performing emergency C-sections to prevent this kind of surgical tissue damage from happening. I was able to have a very constructive debriefing with the obstetrician who delivered my son. We will never know if the scarring was caused by my body reacting to the surgical tissue damage or if she in fact caused it when removing the placenta and swiping the inside of my uterus afterwards. Now, all of that does not matter. I cannot change it, but I managed to educate my obstetrician who promised she would be more aware and tell the women who had emergency C-sections to be cognizant of the warning signs that could indicate Asherman's. I am thankful to and full of gratitude to the doctor who delivered my son by C-section. My son is a healthy boy and this is only because he was delivered quickly. I know that in my case the C-section was a lifesaving surgery. I just wish I had been warned about this "rare condition".

Also, I want to thank Poly and a few special women on the UK Asherman's support group. I had to leave the support group to regain my sanity and I do not think I can return to it again without feeling too much grief by it all. But I want them to know that I admire them and wish all of them the best of luck and a happy and healthy life, with or without their own or more children.

26. AMANDA

My daughter Amelia was born in November 2007, when I was 32. She was our first pregnancy, conceived after just three cycles of trying. It was a good pregnancy, but was unfortunately complicated by severe nausea and vomiting throughout, gestational diabetes, and two bleeds, one of which led to her premature birth at 36 weeks and 3 days. These were uncomfortable, and a little annoying, but as long as my baby was okay, I wasn't too worried.

I strongly desired a natural childbirth, and no medicines including the injection to facilitate birthing the placenta, and the birth went to plan. I delivered the placenta naturally, although I was surprised at how painful it was. I thought after the baby, it would be easy. It did come out with just my pushing, and quite quickly, with no traction of the cord required. The midwife with me was very cynical about my plan to birth it naturally, and I do remember her suspiciously checking the placenta over to make sure it was complete. The on-call obstetrician was happy with the process, so I assumed it was all okay.

Afterwards I had very little milk supply, and at 10 days old, we discovered Amelia was still losing weight. I was instructed to breastfeed, express milk, and formula feed, in the hopes that I could continue to breastfeed. At 8 weeks, due to ongoing bleeding, my obstetrician did an ultrasound, and it was discovered that I had some retained placenta.

I will always wonder if the retained tissue was because I birthed the placenta naturally, without the injection of synthetic oxytocin. There is conflicting evidence on this subject, and some studies support natural placental delivery even if you have previously had retained placenta. I cannot know if I did the wrong thing in this regard.

Due to my feeding problems, and Amelia's ongoing weight concerns, my obstetrician decided to do a D&C, and at the time I was pleased with the decision. I wasn't warned about Asherman's Syndrome being a possible outcome, but I truly feel it was an uncommon result (my obstetrician says she has seen only two cases of AS in her long career). The week after the curettage, my milk supply increased dramatically, and Amelia's weight skyrocketed, so the benefits for me were definitely positive.

Perhaps if it happened again to someone I knew that had retained placenta, I would suggest a hysteroscopy to remove it, so it wasn't a blind procedure. Of course, at the time I didn't know that hysteroscopy was an option.

I continued to breastfeed Amelia until she was 18 months old. My periods never resumed, but I assumed it was due to the breastfeeding. My husband often suggested we should look in to this, but I didn't think anything was wrong.

By 15 months postpartum, I started to notice pain, a lot like labor pains, which would occur intermittently. I asked my GP and she sent me for an ultrasound, which I chose to do during a day I had pain. The ultrasound showed nothing wrong, although it did show my uterus had an open cavity. As the report said nothing was wrong, I proceeded for a few more months before I became even more concerned. For some time, I think I was in denial that anything was wrong, but as the pain was increasing, and I still wasn't having a period, I knew I had to look into it.

I ended up on a Wikipedia page about D&C and it had a brief comment about Asherman's Syndrome being a side effect, so I followed the link and ended up at www.ashermans.org. After reading through the site, I felt sure I had Asherman's, and emailed the site's highly recommended Australian doctor late on a Saturday night. He normally works in Sydney, but despite being in North America at a conference, he emailed me back the next day to confirm that he also thought I might have AS and that a hysteroscopy would be the next step.

I then spoke to my obstetrician, and she booked me in for a hysteroscopy and D&C the following week. Of course, I knew another D&C would be wrong, and so I insisted she only do a diagnostic hysteroscopy.
It was evident that I had scarring at my cervix, which she chose to break through; however, the balance of my uterus was scar free.

I then saw the Asherman's specialist a few days later for a consultation, and he confirmed that my obstetrician had done everything correctly, and if I got a period in a few weeks, all would be well.

As expected, I had that period, the first since I had Amelia, and we proceeded to try to conceive again. We were successful, again on our third cycle; however I had bleeding or spotting virtually all of the time. I had hCG levels taken at 5 weeks, and three subsequent levels, all of which appeared good and increased as expected.

The bleeding continued on and off, but I put it down to a post Asherman's pregnancy, as ultrasound scans at 6, 7 and 8 weeks all appeared okay.

Sadly, at 8 weeks and 2 days in the pregnancy, and on the afternoon of my daughter's second birthday party, I had a sudden flow of blood. We headed straight to the public hospital emergency room, as we assumed I was miscarrying. We usually see our obstetrician at the nearby private hospital, but they do not attend to early pregnancy emergencies there, which meant we did not receive treatment from her, but from the obstetrician on call. The emergency department reviewed my concerns, observed my low blood pressure and ongoing bleeding, and decided to transfer me immediately to the antenatal ward. I was thankful for this, as being in the emergency ward, watched by all of the other patients, whilst bleeding made me feel very uncomfortable.

When we arrived at the antenatal ward, the registrar did an ultrasound, and the baby was still doing well. The heartbeat was slow, but regular, and no-one seemed to know what was causing the clotting and bleeding. Although my obstetrician doesn't work at the public hospital she was liaising with the on-call obstetrician. They decided to monitor me for blood loss, because the baby appeared okay; and we were concerned that if they did anything, that it might cause the return of my AS.

Eventually, after 24 hours in hospital, I was sent for a specialist ultrasound and the sonographer told me I had become priority number one in the hospital. This was of concern, but good to know we were finally being looked after.

I was sent to surgery to see if they could stop the bleeding. I told the house surgeon my priority list was to stem the bleeding, terminate the pregnancy only if they couldn't control the bleeding any other way; to preserve my uterus, but most importantly, to ensure I was still around to be a mother to Amelia, and a wife to my husband. In hindsight, I believe the house obstetrician had no idea what was causing the bleeding. I think she was just concerned to get in to the operating theatre and have a look. My husband and I are pleased that I gave her a priority list, as we are unsure what the outcome may have been, had we not.

During the subsequent surgery, I very nearly bled out on the operating table. Unfortunately, the surgeon had to terminate our baby, via suction curettage, as she thought this might stop the bleeding. Sadly, I continued to hemorrhage anyway, and so I was given seven units of blood, fresh frozen plasma, as well as ergometrine, misoprostol and syntocinon (synthetic oxytocin). Eventually the surgeon inserted a catheter balloon into my uterus and expanded it with fluid to put pressure on the uterine walls, and this stopped the bleeding.

Great detail of my care in this hospital is unnecessary, but it was very poor, and failed to address the cause of the bleeding. Communication with the obstetrician who performed my surgery was inadequate and too slow, the nursing and medical staff showed very little empathy for my loss, and I was sent home without any answers. Suffice to say, I was eventually told I was experiencing Disseminated Intravascular Coagulopathy (DIC) which means that I had bled so much my blood could no longer clot properly, and this is what almost killed me.

Since my stay at this public hospital, the Health Minister in the Territory in which I live has had considerable complaints from the medical and nursing staff, and internal and external investigations of the hospital are being undertaken. I have given my information to the investigators, in the hope of avoiding such poor care for any other women, and achieving an improvement of the obstetric outcomes.

In the following weeks and months, I experienced post-traumatic stress disorder. I chose to deal with that through extensive sessions with a psychologist, and determination to find the cause of the hemorrhage.

The Asherman's specialist felt it was not caused by my AS. He wondered if the placenta had implanted over the cervix and caused the bleed, but wasn't convinced of this. Later we discovered the implantation site was at the isthmus of the cervix, so there may have been something to support this idea, but it is unknown.

Then I spoke to my obstetrician, who suggested it was an arteriovenous malformation (AVM). But when I looked in to this online, AVMs are listed as occurring in the brain and cause headache, epilepsy, and other symptoms, none of which sounded like my issue, so I put it out of my mind.

The head of the maternal-fetal medicine unit pondered a bleeding disorder, called von Willebrands Disease (vWD), or an AVM in the uterus. He sent me to a hematologist who diagnosed me with vWD, but it is only a mild variant which usually causes only bruising, bleeding gums, and heavy periods, which I have never experienced. His belief was that I had a very severe response to the bleeding, but his opinion was that the hemorrhage was still gynecologically related, and my OB/GYN doctors should keep looking.

So, in true Asherman's patient style, I kept searching. I eventually found a radiologist who specializes in AVMs, once I started searching online for AVM and uterus. He referred me for an MRI and an ultrasound to diagnose this rare condition. Only recently, I have discovered I do have an AVM. It likely caused the hemorrhage, and to treat it now requires embolization of the arteries in my uterus, or as a worst case scenario, a hysterectomy. I am yet to ascertain if it is safe to conceive following treatment of the AVM. My priority is to have it treated.

Of course, during this recovery time, I discovered my AS had returned. I was again experiencing very strong cyclical pain, with no bleeding, and so I ended up back at my AS doctor for another hysteroscopy. Fortunately, it is again only at my cervix, and he initially expected one hysteroscopy would fix it, but it appears this has not been the case. I have recently returned for another hysteroscopy, this time with the insertion of a stent, to try to keep the cervix open. My local obstetrician has just removed the stent, and I am waiting to see if the scarring has returned.

It feels unusual to have arrived at this point. I have survived a life or death situation, I have climbed out of my heavy depression, although I seem to fall in to it again very easily and quickly, and now have three diagnoses.

It is a truly rare thing to have an AVM in the uterus, uncommon to get

AS, and von Willebrand's disorder, although relatively common, rarely presents in the severity of mine. I think that to some doctors I am too difficult to fathom, and to specialists in their respective fields, I am extremely interesting. This had made the long diagnostic and recovery process easy at times, and difficult at others.

Where to now? I am waiting to see if my AS has been successfully treated, and my radiologist will attempt to address my AVM very soon. Soon, I hope to be "fixed": back in the condition I was before I started trying to conceive.

Now, though, we need to decide where to from here? Do we have more children, or do we not?

I had initially wanted to have two pregnancies, with whatever number of babies that led to. I have a family history of twins, so it was more about me wanting to experience pregnancy more than once, than the number of babies it might result in. Once I had Amelia, I even thought of maybe a third attempt.

Right now, I have come to a place where I strongly believe that I am not having more children. I have one beautiful daughter, and she can be enough. I feel the risks of a subsequent pregnancy are not only high for a baby during a post AS pregnancy complicated by vWD and AVM, but very high risk for my own life. I am not sure trying to get pregnant and thus putting my own life at risk is a good idea. My obstetrician has told me that if I want to try again, she will support me through the pregnancy, and with the diagnoses we are better armed to prevent a similar outcome. However, I still feel that my family needs me more than I need to risk everything for the possibility of more children.

My husband and I have discussed adoption and surrogacy, and we don't feel it is for us. Adoption is very difficult and expensive in Australia, whether adopting locally or internationally. We don't have the funds to provide for the medical expenses of a surrogate but I also feel if we have more children, they should be our own, carried by me, and if we can't do that, then I don't want or need to seek alternative options. I accept this is not what everyone chooses, but it is right for us.

I am a fortunate woman in many ways: I have a good husband, an adorable daughter, family and friends who love me, and I would prefer to be here to enjoy all of those people than to place my life at risk for the optimistic dream of more children. In this regard, Asherman's Syndrome has changed the path of my life, and where I dreamed it might take me.

27. SONIA

My journey with infertility started five years ago. In 2004, as a newly married couple, and after six months of trying to conceive, my husband and I discovered that he had male factor infertility. In layman's terms, this means that my husband has severe sperm issues that are twofold: first, he has extremely low to absent number of sperm, as well as high DNA fragmentation, which puts me at greater risk for miscarriage. These sperm issues also mean that conceiving naturally would be next to impossible for us.

After recovering from the shock of this initial diagnosis, and after coming to the realization that In Vitro Fertilization (IVF) was the only means available to us to conceive a child of our own, we began a rollercoaster journey of fertility treatments. Over the course of three years, I went through three IVF cycles and was finally able to conceive twins in September of 2008. Unfortunately, at 11 weeks and nearing the end of the first trimester, I was told that my pregnancy was not viable. The twins' amniotic sacs had stopped developing, and no heartbeats were heard during a routine ultrasound scan.

My options for terminating the pregnancy were to follow the natural route, and see if my body could expel the pregnancy on its own. I was also given the option of having a medically assisted miscarriage with misoprostol, a drug used more frequently now for medical terminations; and lastly, dilation and curettage (D&C).

Like many women who have suffered a pregnancy loss, I wanted the whole ordeal to be over with as soon as possible. I had heard that a D&C was both a common and routine surgical procedure, as well as the fastest way to terminate a pregnancy ending in miscarriage. At the time, having a D&C seemed like the best choice for me. In hindsight, I probably should have done more research about the risks of a D&C, although it is likely that I really wouldn't have found out about the reality of Asherman's Syndrome. This is because most references to its rate of occurrence, that I am aware of, are always noted as rare or associated with multiple D&Cs. Because I have never had any issues with my menstrual cycle, or responses to IVF treatment, and this being my first D&C, I thought my risk was very low. But since my own diagnosis, I have met more women who developed this condition after only one D&C.

At the time of my miscarriage, I was being treated by two doctors; one was my fertility specialist, whom I saw regularly during four years of IVF treatments. The other was the obstetrics and gynecology (OB/GYN) specialist to whom I had been referred for my twin pregnancy. In all fairness to these two doctors, I was told about the risks of scarring before I underwent the D&C procedure, and that scarring may lead to infertility. And yet, I was also told that the risk was very low. In fact, the term, "Asherman's Syndrome" was never mentioned. Not knowing what Asherman's Syndrome was at the time, I would have never thought to ask. And after four years of dealing with infertility, and knowing that this third cycle was likely our last, I thought the risks for scarring were low enough that deciding upon a medical termination with misoprostol, or trying the natural route, wouldn't outweigh the benefits of getting it all over with after a quick D&C. I was wrong.

Once I had decided to have the D&C, I did not want to wait the extra week to have my own OB/GYN perform the procedure, but opted to have it done right away at the hospital out-patient care center where my doctor was affiliated. When I awoke from the anesthesia in the hospital after the D&C was finished, I was in pain, and asked the attending nurse for some painkillers. I didn't know it at the time, but this was most likely the first sign that something wasn't completely right after the procedure. Although I expected there to be some discomfort, I felt very strong pain, and the nurse gave me pain medication to relieve it. After more than half an hour, the pain continued, followed by cramping, and I was offered even more medication. I decided to forego the extra medications, in the hopes that giving myself time would help me heal. In the meantime, I was still discharged from the hospital, recovering with little bleeding and only a little discomfort; but I suffered periodically from very strong cramps, which I assumed were caused by my uterus contracting post pregnancy.

Again, I was mistaken; when I didn't get my period eight weeks after the D&C, but instead started having very strong period-like cramping, with no bleeding, I knew that something was wrong. So I followed-up again with my OB/GYN who had me try the progesterone hormone drug, Provera, for 10 days, in an attempt to induce my period. This was unsuccessful.

In the meantime, my doctor also requisitioned some blood work to ensure that my hormone levels were normal, as well as conducting a painful and unsuccessful sonohysterogram (SHG), which is a procedure that distends the uterus and injects saline solution into the uterine cavity to detect scarring or anomalies. This was the point when my doctor told me that I likely have Asherman's Syndrome, and that I would need surgery for the removal of uterine adhesions followed by the insertion of an intrauterine device (IUD) and hormone replacement therapy (HRT). I left my doctor's office in shock. I could barely hold back my tears long enough to get to the car and call my husband. I had already gone through a lot of emotional rollercoaster rides with IVF; but somehow the diagnosis of Asherman's Syndrome following what was one of the hardest times of my life—losing twins—seemed so cruel and unfair. The whole time that we were trying to get pregnant, my fertility was never held in question. Now this had been taken away from me, too.

I immediately began research about Asherman's Syndrome, and found the Asherman's online support group, which is a lifeline of support that I still cling to, even today. While I didn't know it at the time, my husband had already started doing research in advance of my diagnosis, and he was actually the one that found this wonderful support group. I'm grateful to him, and I'm also appreciative that he, too, followed his instincts to look for information when we both knew that something didn't seem right after my D&C.

Through the group, I was able to find the information that I needed to contact the right doctor to treat my condition. Although the OB/GYN who had been treating me was very informed and supportive, I wanted to see an "A lister," the top recommended doctor in Toronto, where I live, before making any more decisions about my fertility. The "A lister" is a doctor who is known for their reputation and skills to treat Asherman's, a specialist that women from the online support group recommend based on their experiences during treatment.

I knew that there were specialists around the world, and particularly in the US, who could help me. However, I really wanted to get my treatment in Canada, where medical procedures are free and where I felt I should be able to get the proper care I needed. I live in this country's biggest city, and I found it hard to believe that I couldn't have Asherman's Syndrome treated by top specialists here. I was also terrified by the thought of flying thousands of miles for treatment outside of Canada, where I had no health insurance and was completely vulnerable, should anything go wrong. This is not to mention the enormous expense for travel and treatment, and the thought of recovering in a hotel room versus the comfort of my home.

After meeting with four different doctors in Toronto, and weighing out all my options, I decided to have my own OB/GYN perform a hysteroscopy to surgically enter my uterus and remove the scarring. I had not come by this decision easily. In the end, I chose not to go with the "A-list" doctor in Toronto because he used a drug protocol which, based on my research, seemed counter-productive for treating Asherman´s. In addition, my OB/GYN was very open to answering questions and very reassuring. He was also the first to diagnose me with Asherman's and had sufficient experience and success in treating it in the past.

And so, in March 2009 I had my first surgery, becoming over-the-moon with happiness when I was told the scarring must have only been in the cervix, and which was likely disrupted, breaking apart when the hysteroscope was inserted into my womb. I had no stent put in, and no hormone treatment, which is frequently required for treating adhesions in the uterus. I was simply told to go home and wait for my period to start again.

But I waited — and waited — for a period that never came. I returned to the doctor for a second round of Provera, followed by a month of birth control pills. I still had no period. I went through yet another SHG to find out why I was not menstruating, even though I still had all the usual pre-menstrual symptoms, including strong cyclic cramping. My OB/GYN was at a loss as to why my menstruation had stopped despite the success of my hysteroscopy. At this point, he recommended consulting with my fertility doctor, because he no longer knew how to treat me.

As I became increasingly aware that my city's top specialists were not even sure what to do, I decided to do my own Internet research on holistic medicine. I felt I had little to lose and much to gain by trying an alternative treatment method, such as Chinese herbs and acupuncture. The acupuncture clinic I chose in Toronto came recommended by specialists who worked in the same clinic as my fertility doctor and provided me with extensive information about Traditional Chinese Medicine (TCM) and TCM accreditation in Canada. While there is still some opposition and reluctance, Canadian fertility doctors are slowly starting to recognize the benefits of alternative approaches to health, particularly from licensed practitioners.

I was prescribed a specific tea that my acupuncturist made out of various herbs and roots, which I drank twice a day, along with acupuncture treatments twice a week. Low and behold, in August 2009 and only one month into the treatment, I finally got my first period.

I felt elated. Doctors were not sure why I got my period. However, it was later confirmed by the A-list doctor I eventually went to see for treatment in California that my second SHG, which was done to check for retrograde menstrual blood flow, likely disrupted the scars, letting some of the blood out. This, combined with the estrogenic properties of the Chinese herbs given by my Chinese medical herbalist, built up my endometrial lining just enough to result in a period.

All seemed well—except for a few questionable cysts that had shown up in my most recent SHG. These were later confirmed by my A-list doctor as benign and nothing to worry about, and which are actually quite common for women my age. And so, I continued with the herbs and acupuncture, having another SHG to investigate these new cysts. In the meantime, I continued menstruating for the next two cycles. While this was a promising sign, my periods became lighter, and more painful, and I had a feeling that my Asherman's issues were not over.

And then, in December 2009, my period stopped again. I had yet another SHG in January 2010, when I was given the diagnosis of "unstuck Asherman's," by my fertility doctor. This is a condition defined by the presence of severe damage to the basil layer, or "root" of the uterus from aggressive or excessive scraping during a D&C. The damage is often so severe that no endometrium can grow back, leaving 'bald patches' of uterine lining. This condition can exist with or without the presence of scars, and is the rarest form of Asherman's Syndrome. It is also untreatable; once the root is damaged there is no more opportunity for re-growth. And yet, the same month of receiving the diagnosis of "unstuck Asherman's" and following my fourth SHG, I had another period. I was then advised to pursue HRT, and have an endometrial biopsy to determine the extent of the uterine damage.

At this point, and after the confusion of different diagnoses from specialists in Toronto, I decided to contact a well-known Asherman's Syndrome expert with a clinic in California who has performed over 1200 procedures to remove uterine scarring. I needed more definite answers from someone who has a solid reputation, and who has also successfully treated two people whom I know personally.

And this is where you find me today. I am writing my story in Toronto's Pearson airport, awaiting my flight to California for yet another hysteroscopy with this Californian specialist. I have stopped all other treatment, except what has been prescribed to me by him. I have decided that the travel and expense is worth being able to finally get some answers, and to provide some resolution to this condition that I have been battling now for over a year.

Unlike many of the other women involved in the Asherman's Syndrome support group, my goal is not to get pregnant—although I would welcome this if it happened. My wonderful husband and I have been through an uphill battle with fertility over the years, and now I have deep battle scars to prove it. In spite of all we have been through, we have come out stronger as individuals, and as a couple. And yet my goal now is for peace and closure, not necessarily to prepare myself for a future pregnancy. I want to have my body function as it was meant to, whether this results in me being able to conceive again, or not.

I believe that the information about the risks associated with Asherman's Syndrome should really emphasize that the possibility of scarring is much greater than previously assumed. The implication that scarring typically happens after repeat procedures, and not a single D&C, provides a false sense of security to women like me, for whom Asherman's can be exceedingly tragic when it occurs following a first unsuccessful pregnancy, endangering all future chances of conceiving. Despite the fact that my final aim may no longer be to have a baby, it is unreasonable for doctors to expect women to undertake surgeries that are actually much more risky than previously thought, without sufficient information to make solid decisions about their care.

I am 39 years old, and I know that my childbearing years are more behind me than ahead of me. This might cause some people to question why I would pursue more treatment if my goal is not to have a baby. My answer to that is that I want back what is rightfully mine: a healthy, normal functioning body, which is always worth the effort, whatever it takes.

Although my husband and I have discussed alternatives to fertility treatments, like adoption, the emotional and financial investment are really more than I feel I can bear right now. My goal is to conserve the strength I need to recover and finally arrive at a place in my life where my thoughts are filled with living, and not always consumed by the issue of fertility. I think I can remember what living with such positive feelings is like. At the very least, I'd like to try to remember what it feels like to live this way again.

I can now imagine myself preparing to close the door on fertility treatment and give both my body and my marriage a chance to move on. But most importantly, what I want is to know with certitude is that I have done whatever is possible in my power to get my healthy body back, so that I can move forward in my life.

Postscript: Since writing my story, I have had my surgery in California, where the doctor discovered that I have ten percent scarring, located mostly in my cervix, and the lower part of my uterus. I now have a stent placed in my uterus to prevent re-scarring, and will continue with HRT, as well as tests to confirm if any scarring has returned after my treatment. My doctor in the U.S. has confirmed that I did not have unstuck Asherman´s, and that my cavity is now 100% open. While such good news has lifted my spirits it has still not changed my mind about pursuing pregnancy in the future.

I think there are times in your life when you need to reconcile with yourself that things will not always happen the way you have planned. I have gone through a lot of challenges and adversity in the pursuit to have children, and I have no regrets. My body, my mind, my marriage, my financial security and my life have all been through tremendous adversity over the past years. I consider it a gift to have all of those things restored to a healthy state. I feel ready to let go, and move on.

Some women might view having a scar-free uterus as an opportunity to try for another pregnancy. I see my new, healed state as an opportunity to shed the emotional hardships I have faced because of infertility, and be grateful for my current health—so much so that I am unwilling to take any more risks. My husband and I have tried everything humanly possible to overcome the infertility hurdles placed before us, and I am no longer willing to destabilize the newfound balance I have with my health, marriage, and financial security for the pursuit of having a child. Sure, I would embrace a future pregnancy with open arms. But it is going to require a little divine intervention—not medical intervention—if it is to happen.

My ending is not yet written, as I have yet to fully complete the treatment for Asherman's Syndrome. But I am confident that all of this will end, despite such challenges ... happily ever after.

28. STACEY

As a child growing up I always dreamed of getting married and having a family. I always loved children and never dreamed my life would take me in this direction. At twenty-seven years old I got married. We spent the first five years of our marriage building our financial stability and buying our first house; soon after we decided to start to have children. We were very blessed to become pregnant with our daughter who is currently eight years old. I loved everything about being pregnant and love being a mom. Shortly after her birth my OB/GYN noticed the placenta did not look complete so he proceeded to do some scraping and said I should be fine. He believed that I would hemorrhage prior to leaving the hospital if there was anything left in my uterus. Everything appeared fine and I brought my baby home after my stay in the hospital. I wondered why the hospital did not conduct a simple ultrasound to check my uterus prior to leaving the hospital but had to assume they were acting in my best interest.

Over the next six weeks I had continued bleeding with large clots and had many conversations and visits with my OB/GYN. The doctor finally listened to me and sent me for an ultrasound which showed I had a 1 lb. retained placenta with a large vein still attached. This would have been life threatening if the placenta had broken away from the uterine wall because it would have caused significant bleeding. The hospital where I received the ultrasound did not want me to leave until they contacted my doctor but they were not able to get a hold of him. Since I had eaten that day they proceeded to schedule the D&C (dilation and curettage) for the following morning. I never felt right going in for that D&C. After the procedure the doctor told me "he scraped as hard as he could and believes it is gone". I asked him if I would be able to have more children and he said "there is no way for me to know." My heart sunk and I left the hospital with the hope that things would be ok. My husband did not hear the comments from the doctor at that time because he was very focused on our six week old baby who needed his attention while the doctor was talking. I believe the doctor said he could not be sure I would have more kids because that day he knew what he did to my body and how hard he had to scrape to remove the placenta. Thinking back I do not see why these types of procedures cannot be completed under the guidance of an ultrasound. With ultrasound you would know the exact location of removal rather than damaging other portions of the uterus.

Things never felt right after the D&C but the distraction of having a beautiful baby girl at home kept my mind clear of any potential problems. I nursed my daughter for nine months which kept me from having any periods. Once I stopped nursing, I never got any periods and consulted my doctor who said it was the pill I was taking. I was not comforted by his treatments so I went ahead and chose a new doctor who could check and make sure I did not have any residual problems from the birth of my daughter. After choosing the doctor he sent me for an HSG (hysterosalpingogram). The HSG is a test that injects die into your uterus while taking X-Ray pictures of the lining. It shows whether or not the endometrial lining is normal or has scar tissue.

At the time I was not terribly anxious and figured everything would work itself out because I felt I was destined to have more children. I later found out that I had Asherman's Syndrome which was stopping my lining from shedding on a monthly basis. At the time I had no idea how serious this condition was and how difficult it would be to cure. The Asherman's was caused by the D&C which removed the placenta. Apparently your body is much more sensitive post birth and it is the worst time to have procedures such as this one.

I depended and trusted in my doctors to know this information and to have my best interest in mind. I have learned not to have these expectations. Knowledge is power even when you are not a doctor.

Even after this diagnosis I thought I would have surgery to correct it and move on with trying to have more children. The doctor said it was easy to fix by having surgery to remove the scar tissue followed by estrogen therapy to thicken and heal the lining. My husband and I were hopeful that this would be an easy fix and we would be moving forward. Our families were behind us even though they were worried that I was entering into surgical options which had their own risks. I was very nervous since I had never had major surgery before but the risks and recovery seemed minimal in comparison with the gift I would receive by having another child.

It was then my surgical life began. I had chosen my first doctor by recommendations and the fact that he was a fertility specialist and OB/GYN. The first surgery was a hysteroscopy which allowed the doctor to vaginally enter the uterus and carefully cut away scar tissue. He started me on estrogen and then repeated the HSG to see progress within a couple of months. The HSG showed a band of scar tissue from the top to the bottom of the uterus. I was willing to live with this but went to a maternal specialist to get his opinion. The maternal specialist said it was a danger to have a pregnancy with the band because the baby could become entangled in it and risk the pregnancy. With this news I was off to a second surgery which was a hysteroscopy with laparoscopy. The added laparoscopy meant they would be making a small incision in my belly button and looking at the outside of the uterus and the ovaries to make sure everything was normal. Following this surgery he inserted a balloon catheter in my uterus to keep it expanded so it would heal on the estrogen therapy. After a week it was removed and the HSG was repeated.

During this HSG the technician was beginning the test and seemed frazzled. He removed the equipment and said I had a perforation in my uterus and needed immediate antibiotics. I was beside myself! How could this have happened? The technician sat down with me and explained where the perforation was. He alluded to the fact that it happened in my last surgery but I later found out that it was impossible since my surgeon had pictures which would have showed the perforation. The technician had made the perforation which caused some internal bleeding and a blood clot near my ovary which took a really long time to resolve. This was a point where my husband and I were at what we thought was our lowest point. It just seemed that nothing would go into a positive direction. It all seemed to just get worse with every attempt to fix it.

At this point I was extremely confused and did not know who to believe. It was time to move on again but this time I moved onto a fertility doctor who strictly focused on fertility problems. I again chose this doctor based on recommendations and location close to home. The new doctor performed the HSG which showed scar tissue which was concentrated on one side of my uterus. He recommended another hysteroscopy with laparoscopy so that he was able to view the blood clot near my ovary and see if he could drain it with a needle. At this point I felt like I was finally in good hands and that all of these problems would soon be resolved. I had the surgery and went on the usual estrogen to build the lining.

After this I started a year of fertility treatments. I chose to start with IUI (Intrauterine Insemination) since this was the protocol that was covered by my insurance and had the least invasive actions. This procedure required the use of a drug (Clomid) that stimulated the ovaries to create multiple eggs. It required a lot of ultrasound monitoring and when the eggs were ready to drop they injected my husband's sperm in past my cervix and hoped for a resulting pregnancy. This was tried multiple times before they recommended that we try the injections of stronger drugs. This was a very stressful treatment because the drugs were not covered under my insurance. The shots were very expensive and completely out of pocket. We had six of these treatments with the last one making nine eggs. They tried to talk me out of the insemination because of the high risk of multiple pregnancies but at this point I had come too far and wanted to take any risk needed to achieve pregnancy. The pregnancy test was once again negative and we were exhausted from the emotional and physical stress.

The next step in the fertility world is IVF (In Vitro Fertilization). This process used the same shots at a stronger dosage but after creating as many eggs as your body would make, they surgically remove the eggs and then add them to the sperm in a lab. The resulting embryos are then transferred into your uterus at just the right time with the hopes of achieving pregnancy. We did not move forward with this fertility treatment because yet again it was not covered by our insurance company. Instead of paying $3,000 for medications, we would be paying up to $30,000 for the entire procedure. I was not comfortable moving forward with this kind of investment not knowing where things stood with my scar tissue and my ability to even carry a child.

When I did not get pregnant I started to do some research which made me realize how serious the problem I had was. At this point I did a lot of research online and found the Asherman's online support group which had documentation of A- List doctors that specialize with treating my condition. I chose one of the doctors and spoke to him on the phone. I sent my records and then began the trek across the county to have a fourth surgery that I was very hopeful would be THE ONE. I flew across the county, met him the same day and had the surgery the next morning. It seems pretty risky as I am explaining this but the desperation for someone to help is so great that you feel you would go to the ends of the earth to fix what is stopping you from fulfilling your dreams.

After waking up from the surgery he explained to me that the damage was much worse than he thought. He read through my prior records and believed that the last fertility doctor had used a laser during my surgery and had completely destroyed most of my lining. Apparently doctors should not be using lasers since the damage can be much more serious if not used with exact precision. He explained that he fixed what he could and was not sure my lining would even have a chance to grow back. He had a balloon catheter inserted to give me the best chances of healing that he could. He left it in for three full weeks which he had never done before but after it was removed I still had scar tissue and missing lining throughout. The thought did cross our mind, at this point, that we should have made the doctor responsible for destroying my fertility but at the time I did not feel that I had the energy to devote to such a negative fight. I wanted all of my energy to be directed in trying to build my family.

Nothing in your life can prepare you to fight so hard and then have continued failure with every move you make. It makes you question your faith, your dreams and life itself. It is at this point that support groups are needed so that you feel that these things are not just happening to you. Many people struggle which results in some failures, some successes, some loss of hope and some realizations that you just need to move on.

I moved on to a new fertility doctor who told me my best chance at having more children was gestational surrogacy. I chose a doctor out of my area (about an hour away) that was highly recommended and had stats online to prove his successes. I was lucky enough to have a good friend offer to be my gestational surrogate and push me into making an appointment for her so she could see what was involved. After a year of preparations, we finally moved forward to do an IVF treatment. We had enough embryos for one try and she became pregnant but lost the pregnancy within two weeks of the transfer. She talked me into trying again with yet another doctor but I was hesitant because the last try cost us $30,000. We found another doctor who we really loved and things were a lot less costly. I ended up with 29 fertilized eggs. We tried two transfers of two embryos each and she did not get pregnant. We were now at 1.5 years and she was emotionally finished. She decided she was done and I was left with 19 frozen embryos in storage.

I do not blame her because she was an angel that stepped in to help me when nobody else could. It was just poor planning and communication on my part that allowed the treatments to go so far to create such a large number of embryos to begin with. This was a hard emotion to balance because I understood the pain she was going through and wanted to support her but I felt very lost and at a dead end since I had no options to carry the 19 embryos I had just created. This situation was what I had always feared because it was not like I could just walk away from fertility now. How do you walk away from 19 living (yet frozen) embryos? They are the babies I am striving for but cannot have them myself. It really makes you feel incompetent as a person and morally you are left with a decision that nobody wants to make. I cannot destroy my embryos and I cannot donate them and always wonder if the children I could not carry were somewhere out there in the world. So every three months my credit card has a charge of $150 for the frozen storage of the babies I can only long for.

Knowing I could not afford anymore fertility treatments or the emotional rollercoaster attached to it, I decided to take a break and look at more options to build my family. At this point six years had passed between surgeries, fertility and surrogacy and we had spent upwards of $70,000. I decided I could not give up on this journey because that meant that all of my hard work and suffering meant nothing. I still did not have another baby and did not have a sibling for my daughter. We started looking into adoption and found a great adoption agency. The cost was slightly less than some other agencies and we liked what they had to say. We started our paperwork but the stress we were under seemed to be worse. After a strong look at our finances and our marriage we decided we needed to stop the journey completely. We were exhausted and had very little in our savings to adopt. We just got to the point where we were sick of struggling. We realized that six years had passed and we had focused on something other than the amazing child we already had.

It is very sad that so many doctors out there do not even know what effect their actions can have on a woman's fertility. I still, to this day, get comments from people that I am lucky to have one child. I agree wholeheartedly that I am lucky to have my child but it does not make it right that my fertility and ability to have more children was stolen from me. My dreams now have to change and focus on what I have instead of what I do not have.

I will always look back on my struggle as a very difficult time in my life but am thankful that I had the Asherman's Syndrome and Surrogacy online support groups to guide me through. I am still in very close contact with some women that have had the same experience as me. Knowing that there are other people out there who understand everything you are going through really makes you feel human again. Moving on has left me with some peace and much sadness. The peace comes from the reduction of stress involved with the disappointments and constant struggling to get something that is supposed to come naturally. The sadness comes from the loss of having the opportunity to experience raising a baby for the second time and when I look at my daughter and see that she will never have a sibling that she can count on for the rest of her life. It is hard knowing that she will be alone in life when we are gone. I can only hope that she will make wonderful friends that will always stand by her side and that I will find complete peace in my heart to live the rest of my life without regrets.

29. Kay

A few months ago, I asked my four-year-old daughter, "What do you want to be when you grow up?" She answered unexpectedly with, "A big sister." My heart sunk.

My father always told me I could be anything I wanted when I grew up. Fighting tears, I replied, "no honey, that's not what I meant. You know, when you grow up, you could be a teacher like mommy, or a contractor like your daddy, or a lawyer like your aunt. You could even be a ballerina, you really like ballet." Now she was upset, "No Mommy, I already *am* a ballerina. I want to be a big sister when I grow up". Well, I still haven't found a way to tell her that I hope for her to be a big sister, too. More than she could ever imagine. More than I could express in words.

My husband and I tried for about half a year to conceive our daughter. Since one of my closest friends was infertile, this was a great fear of mine. Although I had no reason to think that anything was wrong with me. I had never been pregnant before. I remember taking pregnancy tests each month. I was so used to seeing negative pregnancy test results. When I saw my gynecologist that December, she told me to stop worrying about it so much. So I did. I decided to start focusing on something else, finishing my PhD. That next month, as luck would have it, I was pregnant! I finally got a positive pregnancy test!

When my daughter was born, it was magical. My husband and I rearranged our lives so that we could meet her needs ourselves, not relying on childcare outside the home. We wanted to do everything we could for her and that included spending a lot of quality time with her. Being new parents, we couldn't believe how much we loved our daughter. No one could have prepared us for the great joy and love she brought into our hearts. Each day, we felt that we loved her more. This great love didn't seem like it could grow any more. How could that be possible? How could we love our daughter so much?

My husband and I started trying to have another baby when our daughter turned one. By trying, I mean we stopped using birth control. We hoped to have several children. So when I found out, two months after my daughter's second birthday, that I had been rendered infertile, due to a postpartum dilation and curettage (D&C), I was devastated. But I don't think that word, or any words really, can express the utter shock, grief, disbelief and betrayal that I felt. I was so overwhelmed. I remember feeling like I had to do *something* to prevent this from happening to one more woman. My doctor had ignored my pleas for help, when I knew that something was very wrong - when the physical pain had consumed my body. My first plea was to find a doctor to help me. My second was to find a way to stop this from happening to other women.

Upon consultation with my new doctor, a world-wide Asherman's expert, I learned that my case was very obvious. That based on the D&C and pathology reports, there had been a large amount of myometrium, or uterine muscle removed. I was told that my uterus would never be normal again. He couldn't put back what had been taken away. This is something that should have been identified immediately. I was never told that my uterus had been mutilated! The day following my D&C, I did not have any discharge. No blood. No tissue. I was never told that this was my body's response to the injury which I had sustained. The scars had started to form immediately, in response to my body's injury. There would have been swelling in response to the injury as well, thus inhibiting any blood from flowing out of my uterus. I was relieved that there wasn't any more blood or tissue coming out. Little did I know then that my relief would be transformed into disbelief and grief with the knowledge that I would gain.

In the months following my diagnosis, I had this visual in my head of my experience. It's a movie. I'm in my bed and I'm tossing and turning, having a nightmare. You know those nightmares where you have no voice, you open your mouth to scream, but no sound comes out ... you're silenced? Well, it's one of those, and above my head, there's a slideshow of images and films. There are dialogues of the lies my doctor told me overlaid with slides ... excerpts from medical literature ... or "the truth". These facts contradict what the doctors told me. This is how I felt for months. This nightmare of contradiction was playing through my head on a day to day basis. It was a nightmare that I couldn't wake up from - because I was living it. Waking up didn't make it go away and unfortunately, I couldn't rewind it and go back in time to erase what had happened. I couldn't seem to turn off the simultaneous conflicting dialogues or the overwhelming sense of being silenced.

I was silenced; my primary OB/GYN doctor hadn't listened to me. I emphatically complained of how terrible my pain was, how I almost passed out, how I sometimes felt like I was in the final stages of labor. My pain tolerance and avoidance of the ER is quite high. To illustrate this, I had only landed in the ER once before, and that was attached to a backboard almost 15 years earlier. I had fractured my back and was admitted for five days. The pain was so intense, that it felt like swords of lightning were going through my spine. I also went through 63 ½ hours of un-medicated labor with my daughter. Does this give you an idea of the pain threshold I have? Oh no, this pain, I was told by my doctor, was considered normal for women who are breastfeeding and who have low estrogen. As long as I knew what was causing the pain, that should put my mind to rest, and I could choose whether or not to take the estrogen or not. I felt like I was losing my mind each month as my trapped period came, and the pressure and pain increased to the point of debilitation. I just kept telling myself that this was normal, as I had been told by my doctor. Not until I was diagnosed, did I understand that the pain that I was experiencing was because the part of my uterus that still had endometrium in it, was still trying to shed every month. So my entire uterus was contracting, yet because the entire lower portion of my uterus was scarred from wall to wall and sealed shut, it was impossible for anything to exit. So the feeling was similar to terrible menstrual cramps, but with a sensation of pressure building up. This pain lasted for five days every month. My body was trying to have a period, but it couldn't.

Furthermore, I discovered, it was also impossible for me to get pregnant at that point, since sperm could not pass into my scarred-shut uterus. Not only did I want the physical pain to stop, but also the emotional pain that came with the thought of never having more children. I hoped that the surgery would take care of the physical pain, but how would my emotional pain be eased? I felt compelled to raise awareness of my medical condition. I had started to do that in small ways, but wondered how I could make a big impact? Eventually this would be part of my path to emotional healing: trying to make the world a better place by raising awareness about Asherman's Syndrome.

Each night, when my husband and daughter would go to bed, I would stay up late, by myself. My stress only fueled this energy. It was as if I was on autopilot and my laptop was the vehicle. I would do multiple things. I frantically read all of the messages on the support group and responded to as many women as possible. Since I hadn't found anyone locally, with the same affliction, I found solace in an online community of international women. These women helped me immensely, and I tried to help them in return. I created and facilitated videos on the ashermans.org YouTube channel and researched any Asherman's Syndrome information I could find.

It is one thing to be so preoccupied with your own medical condition. I was preoccupied. I am still. But this isn't enough. It's not enough to be so focused on yourself and your own loss. I felt this in an overwhelming way. I had to take what happened to me, and I had to do something with it. I had no control over what had happened to me. I had some control over seeking and getting the best treatment that I could possibly get. But I had more control over doing something proactive. I could research and write: I could help other women. So that is what I did.

I felt like I had been blindsided. I had based all of my decisions on the information my doctor had told me. I felt I had to give other women the information that I didn't get from my doctor. I decided that there needed to be a website specifically devoted to preventing women from getting Asherman's Syndrome, or at least helping them get the information they needed to help with a timely diagnosis. And since 90% of AS cases are caused from D&Cs, I decided to create a website that would meet this need. So I created a website, Dilation and Curettage: Current Information www.DandCnow.info for this purpose. I spent hundreds of hours researching, writing and editing this website.

When I first started this journey, I didn't think I'd have more than two hysteroscopies. At the time, I had read about women having as many as seven hysteroscopies. I just couldn't imagine putting myself through all of that. But I am now part of that club, as I've had seven hysteroscopies and two HSGs. Each time I re-scarred, I felt like my future children had been stolen from me all over again. The only way to stop that feeling - to try to bring my future children, my destiny, back into this world - was to have another surgery and keep the hope alive.

Many hold hope up a great ideal, a noble aspiration - that somehow if you hold onto hope, you're a stronger person. After grasping hope with clenched fingers for over two years, I now realize that hope is something that you put into an empty place inside. But it doesn't fill that space. It just prolongs and lengthens the pain. I have decided that it's a form of self-delusion and self-torture. When I stopped putting so much energy into hope: I was able to let go. Hope gives the illusion of control. Letting go recognizes this illusion. I don't have any control over my infertility whether I have hope or not. The reality is: there is a very slim chance (about 7%), that I will have another child. Hoping that I will have another baby does not increase this chance, and letting go of it does not diminish this chance. Hope is something that you keep when you don't have anything tangible to hold onto. Being on the other side of the fence, I now believe that it takes more strength to let go of hope, yet recognize that hope still exists.

I didn't understand this process of hope, and how it manifested itself through images, until almost a year after I painted my "Paloma Blanca" painting. I painted this following my second surgery, which was deemed successful, so at this point there was a real hope, or possibility, of having another child. Paloma Blanca is Spanish for "white dove" and it was a name that I liked, and had considered for our daughter. The most significant aspects of this painting, are that when I started painting it, I painted a very dark red cross in the center of the painting. This cross is now an under-layer and it's mainly covered by other layers of paint to the viewer. The white dove that flies in the center of the painting is transparent. However, the meaning of this wasn't obvious to me at first.

One day, as I sat staring at this painting with my husband, we realized that the see-through white dove was our dream of our future child, yet it was elusive, a hope, a dream. My husband then mentioned the death poem that he wrote when his uncle died. In it, the white dove is what death is born into, and it flies away up to the heavens. I realized that I had painted the death of my unborn children, the death of our family dream, the death of our hope for the future, on top of a cross: the cross which represented our suffering.

Following my second surgery, I had a diagnostic hysteroscopy, which showed that my scarring had gone down from 60% to about 10%. I was given the clear to try to conceive! I started having some signs that my scarring had returned. A few months after being given the all clear, I found out that my scarring had in fact returned to 60%. With that knowledge, my intense suffering returned as well. I felt like I needed to have a funeral for my unborn children. It didn't help that my doctor told me how great all of my hormone levels were, and that my ovary follicles looked "so fertile". The prevailing, yet undermining fact about my fertility, was that when he looked inside my uterus with the hysteroscope my uterus was over half full of dense adhesions, and it was clearly a view of an unfit womb. To make matters worse, we found out an hour later, that the one tube that had been open, was now partially blocked. Between the blocked left tube, and the partially blocked right tube, I was set up for potentially life threatening ectopic pregnancies. In every way, I was fertile. Except for the most critical, the physical state of my scar inhabited womb.

Is it ironic or symbolic that it was launched following my 9th and final procedure, when I was told by both of my doctors that it looked like I would just keep re-scarring.

So here's where my desperation really came in. Both of my doctors (one who is a world-wide specialist in the treatment, and the other who is a local doctor who has some experience with AS) thought that I might re-scar. We had to come up with another option for this next surgery, since they both believed that I would re-scar after it, but not right away. So the plan was, to have the hysteroscopy and insert a Cook Balloon which would stay in for three weeks, then the week following its removal, I would go to my local doctor for a follow-up hysteroscopy. We were hoping that this would just be diagnostic, to see if the scars had reformed yet, and if they had, they would probably just be filmy, since the Cook had been removed the week before. We had discussed using some sort of assisted reproduction technique, following that procedure, yet I hadn't yet come to terms with that idea anyway. Most pressingly, the idea was to become pregnant as soon as possible, so that my uterus wouldn't have a chance to re-scar. So, the day came for my follow-up hysteroscopy. My doctor told me that I looked nervous, and I told him that in fact I was. I was nervous because I wasn't sure how my uterus was going to look. I had fought so hard already. During the preceding 17 months, I had gone through eight procedures already, and this was my ninth. I was awake for this procedure, and as my doctor put the scope in, I held my breath. Although I could see on the monitor that there were adhesions, I still asked him how he thought it looked. He said that he was surprised by how dense the adhesions looked already (only a week from the removal of the physical barrier). He asked if I wanted him to try to cut them with the micro scissors. I paused. I didn't have any fight left in me. I decided to let him cut for a while and that's when he knew, that the scars were already dense. He wanted to make a few snips to see how much progress he could make. Due to my emotional state, I almost started to cry, and I asked him to please stop. Since they had grown back so quickly, how could I go on? I was so tired of having procedures. I was so tired of the waiting: waiting for the surgery, having the surgery, taking the antibiotics and waiting weeks for the splint removal, taking the estrogen and waiting several more weeks, or months, for the follow-up diagnostic tests - all the while actively hoping and praying that the scars wouldn't return. Why keep fighting if both doctors have told me that they both think that I am just going to keep re-scarring? I felt like this had all been so hard and so long. There was no success in this route. I needed for the next step to come easily. Nothing had been easy so far. Something just needed to happen.

> God, Grant me the serenity to accept the things I cannot change,
> The courage to change the things I can,
> And the wisdom to know the difference.

When I found out that I had re-scarred again, I had to deal with that emotionally in a different way. I couldn't go through more surgeries, now I realized that I would just keep re-scarring. While it was possible to get pregnant, the risks from pregnancy to birth would be so great. In order to deal with this great renewed loss, I did several things. The first thing that I did, was to take a family trip abroad, to distract myself. I had always loved travel. I was distracted by adventure and beauty when I was away. But when I returned, I returned to reality and found myself crying again, every day. My next step in the denial game was that I tried to convince myself that I would be fine with only one child. I told myself that my daughter was enough and that I would just focus all of my energy on her (which I was already doing), and think about all of the benefits of having an only child. I also felt like I needed to withdraw from doing Asherman's awareness work on a regular basis. When I gave so much energy working on projects, I felt like it was taking away from time with my husband and daughter. It also didn't allow me to live in denial very well. So I pulled back, and stopped working on projects for a while. But that didn't help either. By living in denial, I may be protecting myself in the short term, but I still feel the pain of my medical condition daily. I realize that living in denial isn't healing my wounds and it's not helping to heal the wounds of the larger world. It's not helping the other women who are suffering from this disease. It's not helping prevent women from getting this disease. It's not helping promote new research, to make progress in diagnosis, and in treating this disease if I live in denial. I realize that I need to continue this process, as painful as it is, of consciously living with Asherman's Syndrome. I need to live it in a way that doesn't allow me to hide it from myself, or from the world. I need to continue to live in an authentic way that will continue the progress of Asherman's awareness. I will continue to suffer, but I will also continue to transform my suffering. This gives me hope. Not hope for myself and my own ability to have more children. But hope that fewer women will lose their children from this disease. I must continue to feel this great injustice, so that I will be propelled to bring about more justice in the world.

Moving on. I don't know if this is what I am doing. I'm not really moving on. I am at a point where I have put all of my energy into nine surgeries and procedures to correct my scarring. But my scars are always there. My scars are deep inside. My scars don't heal. You can never really get rid of them. They can always come back. When I was at my grandmother's side as she was dying, I said the prayers of the rosary over and over to comfort her, "blessed art thou amongst women, and blessed is the fruit of thy womb".

My final major surgery to attempt to correct my severe AS was in March of 2009. I just had to stop. I couldn't keep putting myself through this, especially when both doctors were telling me that I'd keep re-scarring. I'd done everything I could. I fought the good fight. I was tired. I decided to stop. That's it. That takes strength and courage to stop - to know that you've done enough - that doing more would be hopeless. There wasn't any hope as far as stopping my scarring from returning. I knew that whatever happened next would have to be easy, because I was tired, so tired.

On my list of the three most important things in life, what I hold nearest and dearest to my heart, that would be: my family, God and my health--in no particular order. What is more precious than your family? What is more precious than your own child? Imagine having that life taken from you. There's a difference between God taking a life and a human taking a life away. One is called natural death and the other … well you know what we call that. God didn't do this. A person did this to me, a person who I trusted to care for me and to "do no harm" to me. How could it be, that the things most essential to my heart and my life, could be taken from me through a medical condition?

Clearly my reproductive health had been damaged. My womb is now unfit to carry life, to carry our unborn children. If I am to get pregnant, there are very severe risks to my baby and myself. Those risks to my baby would be: miscarriage, preterm birth, potential intrauterine growth restriction (IUGR) and limb deformity from the scar tissue. To myself, I am at great risk for ectopic pregnancy, due to my one blocked tube and the other partially blocked tube. I am also at great risk for placental attachment issues, including placenta accreta (and its variants). This is where the placenta invades too deeply into the uterus and can cause life threatening hemorrhage during the birth. I could die trying to have another baby. My baby could die. So my health is clearly impacted. My ability to be a co-creator with God - to grow, nourish and carry a child, as she develops her physical body, to enter our world - this has been taken from me. My ability to carry on my family's lineage, my link to my past and thus my future: has been taken from me. But most importantly, my ability to bear my and my husband's child, to bear a sister or brother for my daughter, a grandchild for my parents: this has been taken from me and my family.

When I first told my grandma what had happened to me, she cried. My grandma was a strong woman. I had only seen my grandma cry one other time, and that was because she missed her deceased husband. She told me that she was sad because children are such blessings, and she was upset that doctors had done this to me. She was a very honest, God fearing woman, and she told me that my daughter was the most beautiful child that she had ever seen. She had pictures of my daughter right next to her favorite chair. There were five of them within her line of sight. Because my daughter, her great-granddaughter lifted her spirits. My daughter is the most precious little angel. I think that because I love her so much, and that she brings me so much joy, that I am able to feel such sadness and grief over the loss of having another child. It is by knowing such great love for my child, that I am able to feel such great sadness over the loss of my other potential children. I never knew how much love I could have for a child, until I had my daughter, and I was amazed that my love grew each day, the more I got to know her. My friends with multiple children tell me that they never imagined that they could love their second and third children as much as they loved their first, but somehow, they do. And that this love isn't shared or split between the children, but it's as if more love is created and these new children get their own love. That we are able to create more children, and in this creation, we are able to create more love. Well, there are two things that bring us close to God: love and suffering. Through my processing, I have said many prayers. One that always brought tears to my eyes is entitled, "Prayer in Time of Personal Illness" and the part that I merged with was, "If I am burdened with suffering, lead me to unite myself to Your Cross, so that my pain and sorrow can bring spiritual benefit to me as well as to others".

I haven't let go of everything. I haven't totally moved on. I don't know if I'll ever be able to. I still see myself having three children. I see my daughter running and playing and holding hands with her siblings. I see me holding them all in my arms. I see them growing up and having children of their own. I see the Irish Wedding Blessing, "May there be children upon the children of your children" being fulfilled, as it was for my grandmothers. The spiritual is in the physical and the physical in the spiritual. What does the womb represent? The womb represents a cave, a primordial home, the home that our ancestors lived in, the home that our offspring will be created in. It's a magical place where creation happens. The creation unfolds following God's plan. The miracle of life takes place inside of our wombs. What do the ovaries represent? I believe they represent our link to our past. Our DNA is held within each egg in our ovaries. Our mitochondrial DNA is our mother line DNA, passed down from our mother's, mother's, mother's, mother's: all of the mothers that came before us. They are our mother's waiting to be expressed. They are our mothers waiting to live again. It is our connection to our past, our link to the past. When a child is created, this is our hope for our future: for our collective future, of our past mothers. Many cultures believe that their ancestors still live on in them - that they are in our blood. We now know that's true. Our ancestors are in our blood. They're in each cell of our body. They're in our DNA. Our children are our hope for the future. They are our legacy.

I know it sounds cliché, but, the children are our future. They represent the collective future of human civilization on the planet. They represent their parents´ and grandparents´ future. We look toward our future generation. When I decided to become a teacher, this is where my desire came from, from wanting to work with children to bring about a brighter future for humanity, to bring about a better life for the children when they are in school. When my daughter was born, my hope for the future was renewed on a more intimate level. With the loss of other future children of my own, my hope for the future has been diminished a bit.

My hope, although diminished, is not completely lost. There is very small chance that I could have a baby. It would be considered a miracle, but it's not impossible. There is a possibility, and when there is possibility, there is hope. But this hope exists and is not tended, as tended hope requires a level of energy which has been extinguished in me.

In fact, I took a pregnancy this month for the first time since I conceived my daughter, over five years ago. I was 32 then, I am now 37. I felt like my period was late. I asked my husband to buy a pregnancy test. I wanted to see if I was pregnant, and I was also worried about an ectopic pregnancy being a possibility, so I would want to get an ultrasound as soon as possible if I tested positive. When he came back out of the grocery store with the bag in hand, our daughter asked what he had. I told her it was like a kind of medicine for me. My husband told her that she might have a little brother or sister. I whispered to him to not start getting her hopes up (or his or mine I thought). Although I had a small sense of hope, I kept telling myself that it was probably going to be negative. I didn't want to be too disappointed. I took the test and waited a few minutes for the result. It spelled it out very clearly for me, "not pregnant". I felt numb. I'd had so many disappointments already. I told my husband the result later that night. He said that he was disappointed, that he had felt excited at the possibility of having another baby, and for our daughter to have a baby brother or sister to play with. It wasn't until the next morning, when we were driving in our car, that my husband placed his hand on my knee. Tears started to fall from my eyes, just like the hope - that had once again fallen from my heart.

I can't completely let go yet. I can't completely move on. We don't know what our future holds. How can I move on from the dream that I've held my whole life ... the dream that I've had since I was a small girl ... the dream of being a mommy and of having children of my own?

Today, my daughter asked me, "Mama, when you were little, did you want to be a mommy to babies when you grew up?" "Why, yes, I did, honey, why do you want to be a mommy when you grow up?" "No, I want to be a big sister to a little baby when I grow up."

30. HEATHER

I can still feel myself sitting on my couch late on the night of April 3rd, 2007 with a primal wailing coming from me as I grieved for the loss of my first child. There was the most astounding thunder and rainfall outside and it felt like the universe was grieving with me.

That night I came home from a doctor appointment empty, rather than with the memory of listening to our baby's heartbeat for the first time. We had our 12-week-appointment for our first pregnancy that day and discovered I had experienced a missed miscarriage. The baby had stopped growing a few weeks earlier and we were told there was no option but a dilation and curettage (D&C), which I underwent a few hours later. In the days that followed, as I was home recovering from the procedure, more emotionally than physically, slowly but surely packages of all the maternity clothes I had just ordered started arriving. I tried to wait to buy them until after the all important milestone of the first trimester, but I was just so hopeful and excited to show off my pregnant belly in these cute clothes. I couldn't wait to see the physical proof that I was pregnant and to tell the world. These packages were a cruel reminder of what was not to be. At the time I lost our child, three of my immediate neighbors were pregnant with their first children. Watching them start their families was a tough reminder of what had happened to us and it was very hard to not say 'Why me?'

When I was considering writing my story, I wanted to be sure it would serve a purpose. I hope that the lessons I have learned can make someone else's journey a little easier. Mine is a story of dashed hopes and profound grief and loneliness, but also of learning to accept that you do not have control and to live in the moment and to enjoy the little things.

Our Story

My husband Cory and I dated for several years before we married in 2005. I was adamant that I did not want children, but Cory did want them. What's amazing to me now is that he married me anyway! Then started the dance, he accepted and even embraced not having children and slowly but surely I changed my mind. Again, Cory was willing to change his feelings and desires for the future and off we were on our journey to become parents. I was so happy that I had seen how wonderful our lives would be as parents and couldn't wait to get started. The plan was to have two children by the time I was 35 (I was 33 at the time). I am both a planner and a bit idealistic, so boy was my world about to be rocked.

Cross Country

I can still picture myself arriving back at work the first day after the miscarriage. I paused at the end of the hallway to my office and those dozens of feet to my cube seemed insurmountable. I took a deep breath and told myself, 'Just walk, get to your cube, you can walk." Asherman's Syndrome and recurrent miscarriage is an incredibly lonely journey. There was no one close to me that understood and it is so hard to watch life continue on as you live in a private hell and pretend you are ok. The grief I felt for the loss of my child was profound and it took years for me to move past it.

After nine months of mourning and the ups and downs of trying to conceive again, we weren't having any luck and discovered I had Asherman's Syndrome. I had a hysterosalpingogram (HSG) and the radiologist mentioned scarring. I remember saying to myself 'That cannot be good'. He wouldn't tell me anything more and I had to wait to speak to my doctor. My obstetrician immediately recommended a hysteroscopy followed by a D&C. I had already done research on the Internet and joined the

Asherman's Support Group and knew some of the basics of what I might be facing and what to consider. I asked my obstetrician where the scarring was and how bad it was and she didn't know. She hadn't even looked at the films! From my research I understood that the extent and location of the scarring is important to know and that the last thing you want to do to treat Asherman's is to perform a D&C - the very thing that caused it in the first place. It was maddening! The Asherman's Support Group is a tremendous resource and helped me find the best possible treatment and the best possible doctor.

I had a phone consultation with a well recommended doctor in California. For us the choice was easy, we were going to Los Angeles. For the cost of travel and for some expenses that insurance didn't cover, we could go to an expert who has performed hundreds of these surgeries. My ability to have children was well worth that. In trying to figure out how much we would pay out of pocket, I discovered the insurance system is a nightmare to navigate. I quickly learned to speak in their terms (you need to know all diagnosis and procedure codes, what the charges will be, and what the allowable charges are). The surgery itself was relatively easy. Our doctor was an amazing person who put us at complete ease and even made us laugh a lot. When I complained of pain even after tons of pain meds, he said that was not surprising as they had to give me enough anesthesia to put an elephant under.

After the surgery, we were waiting for a taxi outside the center on the streets of Los Angeles when I realized I was going to throw up. The scene was priceless: I looked like a dog that is going to throw up, weaving around trying to figure out where to go (there was nothing but concrete and some planters). The nurse just looked horrified and Cory looked like deer in headlights as he was trying to shield me from the view of cars passing in the street and find me a place to throw up. The choice was clear and I fertilized the center's lovely planters.

My experience after the surgery was not terrible, but I was in a lot of pain from the uterine stent for the next several days. When I remember that adventure, the first thing I think of is throwing up in the landscaping and how funny that was. I am learning to appreciate the little things and experience joy wherever I can get it.

Two More

After the surgery, the scarring was gone, but my uterine lining was quite thin and I was referred to a fertility specialist. I have always felt out of place at the fertility clinic since I am not going through intrauterine insemination or in vitro fertilization. I don't quite fit in with their usual protocols. But the benefits of easy scheduling, timely and detailed information, and a dedicated nurse (who emails!) have been tremendous. It's the little things that make this journey easier.

I got pregnant the second time with the help of estrogen to boost my lining, but after seeing a heartbeat, we had another loss. I seem to hold on to pregnancies and had to take misoprostol a few weeks later to resolve this one. A few months later we conceived again, but it never progressed and the same thing happened a year later. One of those I was able to resolve naturally and for the other I had to take misoprostol again. My experiences with misoprostol were vastly different in the two instances. The first involved unreal pain and so much bleeding that I had to go to the hospital, while the other was no worse than a bad period. I would not hesitate to take it again if needed; it is well worth it to avoid surgery.

Jealousy

Whenever I encounter a pregnant person or find out someone around me is now pregnant, it feels like a slap in the face. It's hard for me to admit that. It is just an uncontrollable reaction and a harsh reminder of my inability to control my destiny. It's a tough thing to explain and one that my husband still struggles to understand. I know this is a common feeling for those struggling with infertility. We aren't bad people and we are truly happy for pregnant people, it's just hard to completely let go of our feelings of disappointment and loss of control.

Love the One You Are With

My husband and I have really struggled through this journey both individually and as a couple. Both of us acted poorly at times and let ourselves and each other down.

Luckily, we learned a lot from it and from each other and our relationship is even stronger now.

If I had any advice to give a partner watching their loved one struggle with infertility and losses, it would be to, when in doubt, just love them and listen. You will often feel helpless and won't know how to react when all you need to do is show that you care and help us feel heard. The other thing is to be patient as you are able to see things your wife cannot. Sometimes you have to find your own way, even if it's obvious to others where you should be. Cory had the hardest time relating to me in the first year or so and it turned out that he was afraid to acknowledge my feelings because he thought it might validate them to the point of giving them more strength. I spent a long time feeling lonely because of that (as did he). Just being heard is freeing. I am so very happy to know that our relationship is stronger than it ever was.

I think what we both regret most is the loss of these past three years. We haven't been living. I suppose we knew that going through it, but it was just so hard with so many unknowns and traumatic situations. We just couldn't live in the moment. Over the past years, I have identified more with my circumstances than with who I truly am. Finally, I am getting it. I am not Asherman's and I am not my losses and I am not what may not be!

This Isn't Fun Anymore

Our fourth pregnancy was just awful. Neither of us was excited. We were so weary and battered but we also just knew this one too was not to be. I don't know how to fix that. I have finally accepted that never will I be pregnant and care free. But we are still working on the balance of being excited and hopeful, yet realistic. The first several weeks of pregnancy for us are torture, just waiting to hear the bad news. My blood tests always come back great, so I don't find out until at least 7 or 8 weeks into the pregnancy that it is not to be. That feels pretty cruel and makes it really hard to be excited when we find out we are pregnant. And then having to deal with my body hanging on to these babies that are not to be for weeks, while wondering if I will re-scar, is exhausting. In my third pregnancy, it took a long time for my pregnancy hormones to go back to normal, so every week I was going to the doctor and being reminded of my failure to succeed for almost three months.

Categories

When I was asked to write this, I was asked to put myself in a category. Am I 'Moving On' or 'Trying to Conceive'. Well, neither. I don't know if our journey to try to have children is over. But I do know I am done living in the past and the future and not being in the present. I am me and I am going to keep working on being happy now and loving myself and the one I am with, my amazing best friend and husband. And I am going to experience joy wherever I can get it.

As I remember sitting on the couch with that primal wailing after our first loss, what's strange is that it actually seems beautiful to me. I got to feel that. I got to be a Mom. Not in the way I wanted to, but I feel lucky. We created four children and I got to carry them inside me and feel unconditional and authentic love for them. That I will carry with me for the rest of my life and beyond. I think that is just beautiful.

31. COBA

Every night I take a Melatonin pill before bed to help with my sleep disorder. A faded old hospital admission sticker is stuck to the side of the bottle. I started off keeping that bottle because I had no idea how to shred the thing, with all its personal information. Then it just became a habit. So every time I get a new bottle of melatonin, I transfer the pills into the old one. But sometimes I find that looking at that sticker flickers me right back to New Year's Eve, 2008: the eye of my personal post-baby hurricane of Asherman's Syndrome and postpartum depression.

The New Year's Party

I am sitting in a crammed, windowless lounge on "2 West." One of the fluorescent lights sounds like a bug zapper on a steady diet of moths. The old TV is shoved in the corner to make room for a bunch of plastic orange chairs onto which many of us are herded, some placidly, some rather like contrary cats. On one of those chairs to my right is a doughy, middle-aged woman, hunched over and giving off the vibe of a chronic insomniac chain-smoker. But with a smile and some make-up, she's the woman I've chatted with at church, or stood behind in line in the Safeway express lane, or honked at when she took too long going at a green light - everyone and no one. Meanwhile, to my left is a Tolkien-orc-sized biker dude, covered in tattoos and skull-studded leather. I'd laugh at the image he makes, if I had it in me: scowling around the room, shifting uncomfortably in the overstuffed, fake leather chair with busted springs, knees up to his chin. Then there's the bird-boned, white-haired, pale-faced grandma with her walker in the couch opposite me, and the incoherently babbling teenaged girl who just used the full tea cup in my hand as a garbage for her used Kleenex. I'm just waiting for the nurses to finish their cheery spiel so I can grab some munchies and go back to my room. I assume that is the procedure for this kind of gathering. This was the 2008 New Year's party on 2 West: a hospital mental ward I'd been checked into the day before. I remember what I was thinking as I sat there, "How on earth did I get here?" Now I see very clearly: it was postpartum depression, combined with Asherman's Syndrome and my own unrealistic expectations of life.

A Bundle of ... Joy?

To look back now is to track my footprints in crisp new snow. How easy it is three years later to spot where I walked straight off the path into the dark, uncharted thicket. Expecting for the first time at 30, I had a healthy pregnancy, though marred by many months of nausea and fatigue that made me a bit depressed. I mentioned this to my doctor, who assured me that it was normal. Little did I know how often in the next few years I was to hear the diagnosis of "normal" for things that were anything but! Three weeks early, my little girl came into the world after six uneventful hours of labor, aided by a doula and at the end an epidural.

Unfortunately my obstetrician was not on call that day so I got some other doctor, who barely had time to come in and cut the cord and was off again to a C-section. Before she left I remember her *yanking at my placenta* and muttering "What a rat's nest." I wasn't too concerned at the time as I listened to my daughter's first cries and wondered to myself "Am I ready for this?" It turned out that I was not - could not - be prepared for what was to come.

Before I even left the hospital, I had an episode of what might be called a breakdown. I was alone in my room breastfeeding my baby, and I was afraid to move from the chair to the plastic bassinet to put her down. I was having visions of her crushed skull as she lay at my feet. I saw her brains scattered around in little blobs and blood everywhere. In my mind, I had hurled her down violently to the hard tile floor. I had killed her, I had killed her, I had killed my own baby. I couldn't get rid of the thought and of the insane sense that this was real and I rocked frantically back and forth, back and forth, waiting for my husband to please get back from breakfast in the cafeteria.

He found me like this, took our baby from me, and helped me to the bathroom where I almost passed out. Over the next hours, he took our daughter out of the room and let me rest, which sadly consisted only of frenzied crying in my bed, as my mind raced like the proverbial hamster on a wheel. The doctor who delivered my daughter came and asked me a few questions, which she said she would report on to the psychiatrist. However, the psychiatrist on call did not come to examine me, only prescribing something over the phone that the nurse refused to give us a side-effect sheet on, except to sneer "The side effects are in a big book and you wouldn't understand it" and "No breastfeeding." I did not take it, wanting to breastfeed and thinking perhaps I was just exhausted and jacked up on the three Tylenol 3s I had been given in 24 hours. Or perhaps it was hallucinations from the sleep disorder that I figured I had, which had never been properly diagnosed. The nurses kept my daughter with them that night so I could sleep and I did feel better the next day. After a visit from a social worker to make sure I was safe to take my baby home, and having my sister come to stay with us to help, we were able to go. Once home, I tried to cope. But what was full of promise swiftly fell to pieces.

When "Normal" Isn't Normal

Being a first-time mom, it can be baffling what happens to your body. Apparently after-pains are normal, especially when you are breastfeeding.

Some level of clots are apparently normal. Fatigue and unstable emotions are normal. But I was in *a lot* of pain from cramps and my emotions were so far off kilter, I wasn't the same person anymore. Thankfully, my husband had planned to be a stay-at-home dad (I worked from home in technical communications) and he had taken over my daughter's care entirely, aside from my breastfeeding of course. After some badgering on our end, my obstetrician got me an appointment to see a psychiatrist - but not until a full four weeks after the birth.

I waited impatiently for this to come, as I continued to have frightening visions, thoughts, and urges that I couldn't extinguish. I was afraid to be alone with my daughter and asked my husband never to leave her with me. All the while, I continued to have so much pain and cramping. One night, I had some large clots and quite a bit of blood, which seemed excessive. I checked my trusty *What to Expect When You're Expecting* book and we went to an ER. I was told I had a bladder infection and was given antibiotics and sent home. Later, still cramping a lot, I went to my own GP, who gave me anti-cramping medicine and booked an ultrasound for a few weeks later, as soon as she could get me in. I never made it to that ultrasound.

The day of my appointment with the psychiatrist - who not surprisingly diagnosed me with serious postpartum depression (PPD) and gave me some medication - I returned home fairly tired, having walked the maze of a vast and unfamiliar hospital for a while to find her office. When I got home, I went to lie down and as soon as I did, I felt a rush of warmth. It felt like the time I went to the ER a couple of weeks before. I ran to the bathroom and there was no way my pad could keep up. I grabbed a bath towel and screamed for my husband. The blood was gushing out of me. My husband called 911 and I lay down, with a second towel, the first sopping with blood already. When the ambulance arrived, the lady paramedic plodded up the sidewalk and upstairs to the bathroom like she was going for a stroll in the park. My husband was beside himself at the point. Then she asked me to put on a pad. I looked at her like she was nuts. A pad? The blood was pouring out! A stupid pad wasn't going to do anything! But my incredibly patient husband dutifully dug one out of the hall closet, which I then put in my blood-soaked underwear, and which was immediately soaked itself. Finally this woman got the picture and let me grab another towel and some sweats to get me down the stairs and into the ambulance.

I was the one losing the blood but my husband looked like there wasn't a drop of his own in his face by the time I got into the ambulance. He was left in that state at home alone with a baby that needed a bottle (I had since stopped breastfeeding because of all the medicine for the cramps and antibiotics, etc.). He got her fed and took the time to clean up the CSI crime scene in our bathroom. Somehow he managed to calm himself down, pack up our daughter, and follow me to the hospital. He found me in an examining room in a lot of pain, passing clots into a bedpan that felt like I had those giant pieces of liver that you can buy in the supermarket squooshing out of me. After he saw that, he started choking up and I think he was overwhelmed with how serious everything looked. I joked at the time with him that after the birth and now all this, the mystery was sure over in our marriage! It helped to laugh.

After quite some time with the odd nurse checking on me, a well-meaning doctor came to "clean up my cervix." It hurt, but made a big difference to stop the clots and bleeding. I had an ultrasound and was then scheduled for a D&C as soon as was possible and left to rest. Another doctor came by to explain the procedure, which he likened to taking a soft straw to suck out the retained placenta, which, I discovered, had been left behind after my daughter was born:

— "Routine surgery," he said.

— "Day surgery," he said.

— "You need to have it to clean away the placenta," he said.

— "Okay," I said.

I had heard of D&Cs before, and had never heard of any complications, so I didn't question the doctor's judgment, not that I was in the frame of mind to do so anyway.

I went for the surgery early in the morning, before my husband arrived with our baby. I remember waking up in the recovery room, feeling like I had to pee and asking for a bedpan. Instead of peeing, I passed copious amounts of blood and giant clots, again. The nurses were concerned enough to page the doctor, who had, joy of joys, gone home. They called my own OB/GYN, who happened to be there. He came to see me, scolding me that *I* had not called him immediately when I had hemorrhaged. As if anyone had told me that was the protocol! I thought once the baby came out, the obstetrician had nothing to do with you anymore. He gave me something to get my uterus cramping to stop the bleeding and came to check me later. Eventually they let me go back to my room and I discovered my husband was worried sick, as the nurses told him it had taken far longer than usual for me to come back. But the next day, I went home, feeling way better physically. I felt that finally, the physical problems were over and I could concentrate on getting better from the PPD.

Unfortunately, getting better from postpartum depression wasn't like healing from any injury I had ever had before. My PPD didn't seem run-of-the-mill. The psychiatrist who had originally seen me was now on maternity leave and no one took over her cases. After four months or so on the medicine, I wasn't getting better. My GP increased the dose, which just created a worse spiral that included daily stints with my sitting in the shower running out the tanks and sobbing my brains out just to ease my agitation. I still did not trust myself around the baby. First I thought about running away. Then I began to think that my husband and daughter would be better off without me altogether; I counted our money to see if we had as much as would be needed for him to stay home with her until kindergarten and romanced the idea of just making the insanity stop. This included rolling a bottle's-worth of Tylenol 3s around in my hands with a big glass of water standing by and lingering dangerously close to busy roads on my daily walks and watching for big trucks. I felt a frightening sense of elation at the idea of stepping off the curb. It was an I-got-the-job, or I-got-engaged, or I-just-won-the-lottery kind of feeling. The things that should have made me happy made me anxious, and the things that should have made me anxious made me happy. My thoughts and emotions were in chaos. Sadly, my life wasn't going to let me deal with only the depression on its own, which was bad enough. But whose life comes in neat little compartments? I was about to have my PPD compounded and made worse by my journey into Asherman's territory.

Discovering Asherman's

Rewind to six weeks after the birth, which was after all the craziness of the D&C: I had my post-natal check up with my obstetrician and he let me go back on the pill. However, after that, my period never seemed to come back. I asked my GP about this many months later, and was told it was normal after having a baby and that it could take a while. So, I waited it out. It's not like I pined to have my period, after all! Still struggling mentally, we were in no shape to consider another child yet, so I was not worried. But after a year, I began to think this could not be normal. My GP who I visited again with my concerns *was unconcerned* and got me to try a different pill. Still no period. She then gave me a hormone challenge of some kind, to try to force a period. Still nothing. She sent me for an ultrasound and booked me back in with my OB/GYN to get the results. Now, I was worried.

I looked up amenorrhea (once I could spell it properly) on the Mayo Clinic website and discovered a possible cause listed way at the bottom as Asherman's Syndrome - something rare, apparently. I got a funny feeling and googled Asherman's. I found the ashermans.org website and my funny feeling turned into one of certainty and dread. The women's stories on this site were so eerily similar to mine! And the explanation of Asherman's involving scarring and web-like adhesions in the uterus that impede endometrial lining and thus impact fertility was both infuriating and numbing. Wouldn't it just be the icing on the cake after all my troubles that now I would also have this Asherman's to boot!?

At my appointment with my OB/GYN, he talked about my D&C and ultrasound and *mumbled* that I might have some "damage to my uterus." "So, Asherman's?" I said. He seemed surprised that I knew about it and agreed that it might be. Then he wanted me to do another six weeks of hormones. I explained I had just done that with my GP and he wanted me to do it again, "Just to make sure." If I still didn't have a period, he said he could do my surgery the week after the hormones. This seemed fishy, as I had read the horror stories of women on the Asherman's site who had trusted and let their OB/GYNs do surgery on them and I wasn't in a trusting mood anymore.

I did not do the hormones, as I had already done that, and those hormones just made my PPD symptoms ragingly worse. Instead, I got all my records and sent them to an A-list doctor in the U.S. from the ashermans.org list. He diagnosed me swiftly with Asherman's, took a good hour to explain it all on the phone in a most kindly and open way, and explained my possible next steps. I booked a surgery and then set out to find someone to take care of our daughter so my husband and I could go. No one was available. And while I struggled to find that help, my husband announced that he couldn't go through all this again. He couldn't face another pregnancy. Given all the potential for post-Asherman's pregnancy complications or miscarriages in addition to the likelihood of another bout of postpartum when I wasn't even over the first bout yet, he didn't want to see me suffer any more or go through the experience of the past year or so again. Could I imagine having a miscarriage and postpartum, and no baby to show for it afterward, he pointed out to me. All very logical, but the emotions that these decisions stirred up in me were consuming. And this is where my world truly fell apart and I spiraled toward that New Year's stint on the mental ward.

Uncovering Unacceptable Expectations

Although I was with a much better psychiatrist at that point, I was reluctant to disclose the full picture of how I felt and what I was experiencing in my daily life. I wasn't hiding anything purposefully; I just didn't have the ability to express negative feelings openly, or the confidence to admit them without a sense of shame or failure. Plus I figured if I thought hard enough that it would be okay, then it would. Several personal crises including the Asherman's, tremendous relationship friction, and a self-injurious incident later (minor but frightening enough to me that I would do anything at all) and I drove myself to the ER for help, my psychiatrist's office unfortunately closed for the holidays. After my three-day stay there on the mental ward, I enrolled in group psycho-educational classes that my psychiatrist recommended. He had previously said I should take them, but I had presumed I could handle things and didn't need them. Boy was I wrong! The classes helped me tremendously with my PPD and led me to uncover underlying ideas about myself that were holding me back and interfering with my recovery.

I imagine that most people have a picture of what their successful self looks like. Like so many women of my generation, my picture was of a happy marriage with at least two or three children and a successful career (in my case, my own home-based communications business) on the side. Piled on top of this was an endless list of ideals - all very positive but also time-consuming. I pictured myself as a woman who was strong enough, capable enough, and committed enough to be able to make time to do all these things, and to do them to the highest standard:

- nurture my marriage relationship with couple-only activities,
- meet all of my husband's emotional and other needs,
- meet all of my kid's physical and learning and entertainment needs,
- create and nourish close friendships of my own and as a couple,
- make a positive impact in my church community,
- pursue opportunities to stimulate my career and creative impulses,
- go to the gym regularly to achieve and maintain the elusive hot bod,
- and (of course!) keep up a cozy house that is clean and homey, where the cat box never smells, laundry is always done, home-made healthy meals are on the table at 6 pm, bills are paid on time, the car is serviced every 5,000 km on the dot, and the snow gets shoveled promptly after it falls.

Somehow, my self-image had mushroomed into this unrealistic superwoman. It was like a painting of a mountain scene with a French cafe squashed into the valley in the middle and still life fruit bowls and flowers in the corners—too much going on. Part Robert Bateman, part Picasso, and part Rembrandt. It just made no sense to look at. But you never really examine your own self-concept until something comes along to mess it up. And for me, it was Asherman's that came calling.

The Tyranny of Maybe

Having Asherman's in combination with my PPD brought the harsh reality of having only one child, not the two or three I had envisioned in that picture. This was quite a cornerstone of my successful self-portrait. And rail against that thought as I did, I could not change my circumstances enough to provide the absolute certainty that I would not put my family through the nightmare that came after the birth of my daughter. Working harder or being more dedicated would not change things. And I was willing to sacrifice my own mental and physical health, but not my husband's or my daughter's.

I was distraught at the thought that I had no control over this aspect of my life: I could not make it a success anymore. It was a failure. I was a failure. I felt *I* had failed to make sure that my placenta came out whole and was properly examined. Maybe if I had hired a midwife instead of a doula, that person would have double-checked on the work of the doctors and nurses. Maybe I should have got out of the bed and checked my own placenta! I do remember reading in the baby books that the placenta needed to come out completely. So really, wasn't it my own fault? I smothered myself with this false guilt. And maybe if I had asked more questions before I let that doctor do a D&C on me at four weeks postpartum, I could have ferreted out more options. And maybe if I had been more forceful with my doctors that no period was *not* actually normal, I could have been treated sooner, before the scarring got too bad. And maybe I could have ignored or suppressed my PPD or pretended it didn't bother me so my husband would not have known and then maybe that wouldn't have become an additional barrier to having more kids.

I knew these were unrealistic thoughts. But I couldn't stop blaming myself for this failure. Then it was as if everything became a failure. I hadn't got back into shape after my pregnancy yet. The renovations in my house were still not done. I wasn't spending enough time with my daughter. I was constantly arguing with my husband about anything and nothing. I wasn't spending much time with friends and was isolating myself from people from church. And I wished I could take on more contract work but felt I didn't have the discipline to do so with my husband and child at home as well.

I began to have trouble making simple decisions. Do I take this contract job? Do I tell my husband I want to go for a holiday? Should I take time off at all? Over time, it got to the point that I found myself standing in front of bakeware in Zellers, and it took me twenty minutes to choose between two medium sized loaf pans. I didn't know who to trust and felt I could not trust myself. It was just an $8 loaf pan! I used to be so confident and optimistic and happy. I felt a hollow spot inside because I simply didn't recognize myself anymore. Other people had let me down, people I had trusted - the doctor who had tugged on my placenta and run off, the well-meaning doctor who "cleaned up" my cervix, the doctor who did the D&C, my first psychiatrist who left me with no one to turn to - and in letting them do this to me I had lost confidence in myself.

Making Sacrifices to Move Forward

It was at this point that I broke down and made my biggest sacrifice and freed myself to move forward to a truly successful and fulfilled life. Just like the women of the 60s throwing their bras in bonfires, I decided to strip away and shed all the false requirements I had gathered to myself as I went through life. It has been as difficult as scraping iron filings off a magnet. These ideas are so firmly fixed in my subconscious; I always want to turn to them to judge myself! But I am working to redefine success and failure by sacrificing my pre-established underlying conceptions of what a successful woman should be. This is a logical, intellectual effort I need to make to make sense of my world and to be able to move on.

People may sneer that this doesn't sound like much of a sacrifice. But basically, I am sacrificing my pride and self-trust. I'm accepting that I no longer need to trust in myself to do everything exactly right. I can let go and trust in God (as I always supposedly did!) to take care of me, whatever my health, whatever my number of children, whatever my career status. I am surrendering my imagined sense of control and rebuilding who I am. Surely, this is no mean feat to be scoffed at. What I am realizing is that I am not, was not, and will not always be in control but that the God I believe in certainly is and with that knowledge I can make the best of what happens in my life with my faith and not my fear at the helm.

Now I feel free to look at what a successful *Coba* should be, given my own personal limitations. And a successful Coba is happy with her loving husband and amazing little girl, who is now so obviously a true bundle of joy and energy, of love and curiosity. I can look at my laundry list of requirements and reframe them:

- I see that taking time to be alone with my husband is good for everyone, but doesn't necessitate elaborate planning and expense and isn't my sole responsibility.
- I realize I am one person who can never meet all of my husband's emotional and other needs and he has to find other people for some things.

- I realize that I can make a huge contribution towards my child's physical and learning and entertainment needs but my husband has a role to play as well.

- I know that I can lean on close friendships for support, not just give support to others.

- I know that at times in life, I will have more time to give at church, and at other times I will receive and there is no failure in receiving instead of giving.

- I understand that work will always be there and have no more angst from putting it on hold for three meager years while my daughter needs my attention, and I see that I can do things to stimulate career and creative impulses in the meantime.

- I recognize that it is hard to make time to go to the gym regularly when I have a little one and that I can do other things to maintain good health - but not to attain some imaginary Photoshopped hot bod.

- And I have noticed that of housework there is no end and no one will die if the cat box smells for a day or two!

Most of all, I have seen in myself that there is no shame in not being able to "have it all" or "do it all" according to some outrageous and unrealistic standard that has seeped into me over time. I have not failed in the family department by accepting that I can have one child instead of many. I have not failed in the career department by accepting that it is okay to take a couple of years off to be with that one child. Every woman has her own journey and circumstances and we do not all have the same destiny. Mine happens to include one amazing child and husband. And now it also includes a happy and fulfilled me, looking eagerly forward to a life once again full of promise. So I think it is time I got rid of that old pill bottle with the sticker reminding me of my New Year's Eve on the mental ward. I can see now that I have learned the lessons I needed from my PPD and Asherman's experiences. I need no more reminders holding me back. It is time to truly move on.

32. JF

Anger can be destructive but it can also fuel constructive changes. I do not see my own struggle with Asherman's as a fateful, spiritual journey needed to bring me closer to God or fill me with a newfound sense of wisdom about life. This outlook would amount to submitting to a system that needs to improve. I will never see my Asherman's as something that was 'meant to be.' I'm an idealist who believes that people need to take action when they see something wrong. Something must be done to raise awareness about Asherman's Syndrome and how miscarriage is managed.

Over the past two years I've read all the medical literature I could about Asherman's, my scientific degree is giving me a unique position to access and understand these technical articles. I hope that by sharing my experience and using my personal and specialized knowledge, I can open people's eyes to the risks of D&Cs being pushed on women when alternatives exist. I also write extensively about Asherman's Syndrome prevention in my blog and YouTube clips.

JF's Story: Stolen choice and a stolen future

I'd left having children until later in life because of my studies (I have three university degrees including the PhD in molecular microbiology) and married at 35. When I was 39 my husband and I had finally settled into jobs, bought a home and were ready to start a family. Perhaps it seems naive, but there was no reason for me to think I would ever have any fertility problems: I was in good health, never had gynecological problems and many women in my family gave birth at my age without problems. I never would have suspected that the actions of a doctor would cause my infertility and so much anguish in my life.

It took only three months for me to conceive but after walking around for eleven weeks in bliss, my husband and I found out at my first ultrasound that there was no embryo development: what is commonly referred to as 'blighted ovum'. I always knew miscarriage was a possibility due to my age but was devastated and shocked to learn that it could happen without any bleeding. My obstetrician wanted to do a D&C as soon as possible to remove the 'products of conception'. But all I could think of was a story I'd read decades ago in my mother's *Good Housekeeping* magazine about a woman who'd had a botched abortion resulting in severe uterine scarring that would prevent her from ever having children. I still recall the grotesque description of uterine tissue hanging out of her vagina. D&Cs seemed an archaic procedure and as my obstetrician answered my questions, a sense of panic came over me. This is where it could all go wrong.

-Yes, he said, D&C is the same procedure used for abortions.

-Yes, D&C for miscarriage entails the same risks as abortion.

-No, the doctor does not use ultrasound or any imaging technique to see what he is scraping.

-Yes, D&C can cause Asherman's Syndrome.

Though I was assured when my obstetrician said that Asherman's was an 'exceedingly rare' occurrence, I was still not convinced. At my age I did not have a lot of time to deal with complications from medical mishaps and was not about to take any chances, however minimal I was told they were. I inquired about alternatives such as medication and waiting for a natural expulsion. My obstetrician said that the drug misoprostol was not 'effective,' especially for a blighted ovum at 11 weeks. I was told that waiting to expel naturally was likely to take weeks and also be ineffective. I didn't question the accuracy of his statements, but intent on avoiding a D&C, I opted to wait. My obstetrician was visibly annoyed by my decision. Three weeks later, my uterus naturally emptied itself. After an ultrasound, my husband and I were very relieved that the expulsion was complete. But my obstetrician wanted me to return a few days later and this time after a simple office scan he decided that I had retained products of conception, an open cervix and 'needed' a D&C.

Again, I was hesitant. I again inquired about using misoprostol and got the same response. Furthermore, he scared me with the possibility of infection, saying now that my cervix had opened there was the possibility that I could acquire an infection if I did not have a D&C and soon. The longer I waited, he said, the higher the risk of infection. He said that I could develop Asherman's Syndrome from an infection even if I did not have a D&C. Today, I know that Asherman's from infection alone is unlikely, and that surgery is as likely to result in infection as natural miscarriage. But since all this information was unknown to me at the time, I was scared enough to accept a D&C a week later. To this day I am pained by regret: If only I never had that D&C. Yet I had tried everything possible to avoid it. I had even tried to get a second opinion but the earliest appointment I could get was three months later, even after I explained my situation. It was the week before Christmas and all the doctors seemed to be busy before the holiday.

When I asked if my doctor could use ultrasound guidance during the D&C to avoid damage, he said it was not possible to accommodate an ultrasound machine in the operating theater. Looking back I'm still bewildered at how insightful my suggestions were, given that I thought of them instinctively. I was given powerful antibiotics as a prophylactic measure against infection to 'prevent' Asherman's Syndrome. Other measures to 'reduce' the possibility of Asherman's were to get my obstetrician to perform the procedure (instead of an inexperienced registrar) and to have it performed using suction. I learned later that none of these preventative measures were proven to be effective in the medical literature. I don't know of anyone else with Asherman's Syndrome who went to such great lengths to try to avoid the procedure. I might be able to accept my situation more readily if the blame were with me rather than with my doctor.

It would be a cruel irony if I were to develop the exact condition that I feared, but after my fateful D&C I suspected something was wrong. I came across Asherman's Syndrome while searching for my symptoms on the Internet. I hoped that my newly painful and scant periods were a sign of something else but there was no denying that these symptoms were a red flag for Asherman's Syndrome. I even felt that because I talked so much about it with my obstetrician prior to having a D&C, I had some sort of guarantee that it would not happen, that he would try to do everything possible to make sure he didn't accidentally scrape too deeply. The doctors I saw didn't believe that I could have AS. Rather, they made me feel like a neurotic hypochondriac.

I joined the Asherman's Syndrome support group before I was even diagnosed. It was the only website at the time that didn't make Asherman's seem like something incredibly rare and nearly impossible to acquire. And there were active discussions about treatment and regaining fertility. The other members didn't make me feel like I was a delusional hypochondriac. I wanted to find out as much as I could about the condition, its correction and which doctors to trust, and as quickly as possible. I had lost all confidence in doctors, feeling so betrayed by my obstetrician. I was afraid to undergo another invasive procedure in case it caused more harm. But I found out there was an excellent specialist in my area and booked an appointment to see him.

I'll always remember the day I had an in-office diagnostic hysteroscopy and was told I had stage III AS, and the melancholic song that played on the car radio on my way home, as I contemplated my future. There was no denying the damage had been done to the basal endometrium, the crucial regenerative layer of the uterine lining. The adhesions were thick and fibrotic and they extended upwards from the right lower quadrant of my uterus. The Asherman's specialist told me to use contraception until my corrective surgery because, although unlikely, if I did get pregnant it could be dangerous for both the baby and me.

Here I was, a 39 year old woman without any children, wanting to start a family, and being blessed with the ability to conceive naturally, and my obstetrician seemed to have thought nothing of risking it all with a surgery I didn't even want or perhaps need to have. Indeed, the pathology report from my D&C mentioned 'no obvious chorionic villi detected'. How easy it had been for him to steal my future and get away with it with no consequences whatsoever. I knew the consensus would believe that I hadn't ever had any fertility, or any left anyway. At my age I appreciated how precious my fertility was, so having it suddenly snatched away was unbearable. I had to wait quite a while to undergo corrective surgery. It's so hard to wait any amount of time when one's biological clock is ticking so loudly. I cried a lot. Having just experienced the enticing prospect of motherhood, the timing of this deprivation and the possibility that it would be permanent tormented me. I have never been a good sleeper and these worries kept me awake at night.

My hysteroscopic adhesiolysis was performed in October 2007. I had a uterine stent for two weeks after the surgery and had two cycles of estrogen therapy. I was hopeful when I learned that my uterus was adhesion-free and got the green light to conceive. A few months after my corrective surgery I decided to resign from my job at a research institute to concentrate on getting pregnant. I knew this was going to be a difficult time emotionally and even if

I was successfully pregnant, it would be a high risk pregnancy with many visits to the obstetrician. I was advised to try to conceive naturally for three months and if unsuccessful, to seek IVF. I hate to admit it, but I felt resentful walking into that fertility clinic. I wouldn't have found myself in this situation if I hadn't had a D&C. People who have never had AS don't really understand it. It doesn't seem to click that AS can happen to anyone, robbing them of their fertility overnight. Of course some people and doctors seemed to think that at my age, infertility was something I was going to experience anyway and AS was just a little glitch in my journey to motherhood. When I hit that magical age of 40 I was supposed to accept that my natural fertility disappeared into thin air. It was like I was Cinderella and my coach turned into a pumpkin because the clock struck midnight! Certainly I knew that I was not as fertile as I would have once been, and that the risks of miscarriage were greatly increased, but I didn't believe that getting pregnant over 40 without IVF would be as close to impossible as they implied. I did two IVF cycles in all. Neither cycle resulted in a pregnancy, with only one extra embryo left over to freeze.

I was extremely frustrated after not falling pregnant during the two years after corrective surgery. I couldn't understand how I could go from fertile to infertile in the space of a year and was convinced a factor related to AS was the underlying cause even though almost no doctor was willing to concur. I slowly started to accept that I might never become pregnant – that even if AS played a role in my unexplained infertility, I would soon face age-related infertility, the boundaries of which were blurring with each other.

To my elation and amazement, two weeks before my 42nd birthday and four months after my last IVF cycle, I fell pregnant naturally. My initial joy was soon replaced by constant worrying. At first I was scared of having another blighted ovum or miscarriage. This time I made sure to have ultrasounds as early and frequently as possible for my peace of mind. I tried to convince myself that this was 'the one'. But I also knew that post AS pregnancies are high risk, with possibilities of placenta accreta, incompetent cervix, growth retardation and premature delivery. At age 42, I was also at an increased risk for having a baby with chromosomal abnormalities. Week after week things progressed well and when we saw the heartbeat at 7 weeks we were overjoyed. It seemed surreal. I relaxed a little knowing the vast majority of pregnancies that make it to this stage would make it through to birth. Then all our hopes came crashing down at our 12 week scan when the screening scan came back with a 1:2 chance of Downs, trisomy 13 and 18. Another test confirmed our worst fears: our baby had died as a result of chromosomal abnormalities at 14 weeks gestation. The saddest part is that while I once hoped to see her little heartbeat, I was relieved when it suddenly disappeared because it saved us from making a painful decision. There was no question of having a D&C. This time around I underwent misoprostol evacuation in hospital, although it needed completion via hysteroscopic removal of retained products a few weeks afterwards.

I couldn't believe it when two months later I was pregnant again. I tried to invest less emotionally in this pregnancy but of course this is not possible. A few days after a heartbeat was detected, I no longer felt pregnant and an ultrasound confirmed that I had a missed miscarriage once again. The implantation site was slightly low and there was poor uterine adaptation after implantation. I will always wonder if the loss was AS related or not. I will also never know why I suddenly got pregnant again after two years. Perhaps my endometrium was still repairing itself from the damage of the D&C? Perhaps the hormones used during IVF contributed in repairing my endometrium? Each time I fell pregnant, I'd feel a great relief that I was going to have at least one child and I would start feeling confident that I may even have a second one - the number I've always wanted. But then I would miscarry and be back to square one: complete uncertainty, a life in limbo. *Just one child*: that would make me eternally grateful.

It breaks my heart when I recall someone saying how much they pity women who never get to experience motherhood, said not out of maliciousness but clumsy honesty. I have watched my nephew, born several years before my Asherman's, grow from an hour old newborn to a family member I love deeply. I am amazed at how much I could love someone who just suddenly appeared and am awed knowing that I would love my own child more than I can imagine. For my doctor to take that potential for this love from me fills me with so much grief, bitterness, and anger I sometimes feel I cannot contain it and will burst. Looking back over the scenario that unfolded was like watching a nightmare in slow motion where I was powerless to act. I have never felt such a sense of impending doom and so compelled to avoid something. I feel like I've been the victim of a genocide where all my future descendants were prevented from ever existing.

On Prevention

The most tragic thing for me it is that I got Asherman's before I ever had the chance to become a mother. This fact drives my motivation for prevention. The single most important thing I've learned from my personal experience: awareness about the risks of D&C is simply not enough; the right to access preventative options such as drugs and hysteroscopy is essential. Over the past two years, the more medical literature I read about Asherman's, the clearer it becomes to me that prevention is being overlooked. It is absurd that so little is being done about prevention when alternatives such as hysteroscopy and drugs like misoprostol are safe, available and highly effective. Yet D&Cs continue to be one of the most common surgeries performed on women of reproductive age and remain standard care for miscarriage in many countries. Why aren't women being at least offered an active option other than D&C? I was a scientist who had informed herself both about AS and alternatives to the D&C and yet I was powerless to get the treatment I wanted.

Few people have heard of Asherman's, and many doctors know little about it (even though they may think otherwise). AS remains underdiagnosed or misdiagnosed and it is often difficult to make the link between a procedure and subsequent complications that may not be detected until much later. AS and D&Cs are often associated with abortion, a highly contentious topic whose moral debate overshadows the issue of D&C safety. Many women find it hard to believe that D&Cs can be harmful because either they have undergone it or they know others who have without any problems.

Two years have passed since I wrote the above. My last hysteroscopic curettage after my second post-Asherman's Syndrome miscarriage was technically difficult. Soon afterwards, I had three more very early miscarriages in close succession. A recent ultrasound suggests I might have Asherman's Syndrome again. My passion for clinical research and evidence-based medicine led me to enroll in a master of science in medicine in Clinical Epidemiology. I thoroughly enjoy it and look forward to using my knowledge and skills in research that is relevant to Asherman's Syndrome. I've learned that local hospitals have recently begun offering medical management of miscarriage and I hope that by sharing my experience on the Internet and with my doctors, I somehow played a part in this. To any woman who might be reading this now and doesn't know how they will face a childless future, know that just like when someone dies, the pain eventually gets less, though you will never forget.

Lastly, I wanted my story to emphasize that treatment is not always successful, and even if it is, sometimes it's too late: I got AS at a very critical stage in my life when my natural fertility was declining and I lost an irretrievable year. Still, I'm grateful for Poly's support group and to the Asherman's Syndrome specialists and the high risk obstetrician I found out about through the group. Without their expert treatment I would not have been able to fall pregnant twice. Although I wish that I could have written this experience with a 'successful' ending, I know that it wouldn't change how I view things, or the message I want to share with other women and doctors: that no woman should ever have to go through what I did because of a routine surgery *for which there are alternatives.*

VI. DOCTORS' PERSPECTIVES

31. PAUL D. INDMAN, M.D.

San Jose, California, USA

DIAGNOSIS AND TREATMENT OF ASHERMAN'S SYNDROME: AN OFFICE BASED APPROACH

My first patient with Asherman's Syndrome (AS) came to me over thirty-five years ago, having made her own diagnosis. This was long before the Internet, and after her doctor failed to recognize the cause her monthly cramping and lack of menstrual periods. After hysteroscopic treatment she was able to have the baby she wanted. I still see her every year and remind her how impressed I was that she made her own diagnosis.

There is much we know about the treatment of AS, and much that we still need to learn. We often use traditional "wisdom" to make medical decisions. There is a move towards "evidence based medicine" where we look at actual clinical studies rather than relying on our perceptions. At times what seems logical may not in fact be correct. One such example is that after major abdominal surgery patients have traditionally been given a liquid diet and then slowly advanced to solid foods. But a study in which half the patients were given the liquids and the other half a regular diet found that recovery was much faster in the group given a regular diet. *So what seems to make sense really needs to be tested and not just assumed.* Some of our knowledge is based on scientific evidence, but it is time consuming and expensive to carry out scientific studies, so many questions about the best way to treat AS remain unanswered. I'll try to emphasize what is based on scientific evidence and what hasn't been scientifically proven.

Two Types of Asherman's Syndrome

Long before vaginal probe ultrasound became a simple office exam I realized that women with a history of monthly cramping with little or no bleeding following a D&C frequently had adhesions localized to the lower portion of the uterus near the cervix, leaving a normal upper portion (Figure 1). Ultrasound often will show normal endometrium in the upper uterus. This is usually easy to treat and has an excellent prognosis. Figures 2a and 2b show the hysteroscopic view of this type of adhesion during and after treatment in my office.

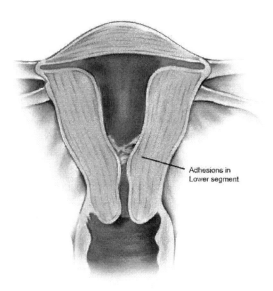

Figure 1: Adhesions in lower uterine segment

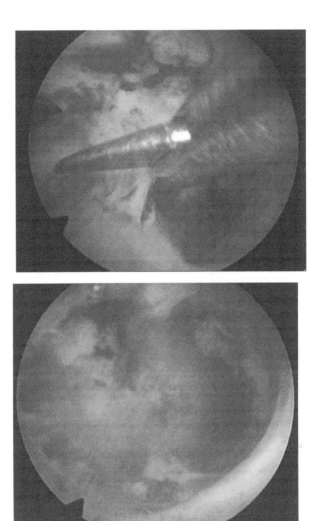

Figures 2a, 2b

Figure 2a: Adhesion in the lower uterine segment being cut with hysteroscopic scissors in my office.

Figure 2b: Normal uterus after cutting adhesions. She subsequently went on to have two normal pregnancies and deliveries with no complications.

Women with little or no cramping, and who have little or no visible endometrium on ultrasound often have adhesions in the upper part of the uterus (Figure 3), and may include the cornual areas (where the fallopian tubes originate). Treatment is far more difficult as the cavity may be entirely obliterated. Mild adhesions and adhesions in the center are easier to treat than adhesions in the cornual areas.

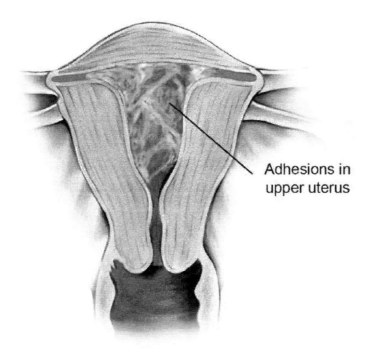

Adhesions in upper uterus

Figure 3: Adhesions involving entire upper uterus

Diagnosis

The "gold standard" for diagnosing AS is hysteroscopy — looking directly into the uterus. While hysterosalpingogram (HSG) and ultrasound with the infusion of saline into the uterus (sonohysterogram, or SHG) can be helpful in outlining the uterine cavity, neither are as sensitive as hysteroscopy in detecting adhesions. If the lower portion of the uterus is blocked then neither HSG nor SHG can tell whether there are adhesions in the upper portion of the uterus.

Hysteroscopy for diagnosis and treatment

Diagnostic hysteroscopy involves placing a thin telescope (hysteroscope) through the cervix and into the uterus. I first numb the cervix (this is easily done and rarely uncomfortable). I attach a video camera to the hysteroscope, so my patient can also see, and then insert the hysteroscope into the uterus under direct vision while using saline to fill the uterus. Then it is possible to see any adhesions directly. Adhesions can be cut with tiny scissors placed through the hysteroscope.

Hysteroscopy in the presence of dense adhesions that entirely block entry into the uterus is more complicated. It's like digging a tunnel through a mountain — how do you know which direction to go without navigation? The use of ultrasound guidance has been a major improvement in treating AS. With the hysteroscope I can see and cut adhesions in front of it, but can't see what is beyond the adhesions. With abdominal ultrasound being done while I am doing the hysteroscopy I can see where I am heading and how close to the top or edge of the uterus I am. That is far more effective than using laparoscopy, which only shows the outside of the uterus. It also avoids the risks and discomfort from laparoscopy. Figures 4a-c show the hysteroscopic view of these types of adhesions.

There is a controversy about what instruments to use to cut the adhesions. Sharp dissection uses tiny scissors placed through the hysteroscope. They cause NO damage to surrounding tissue. Other instruments use laser or electrical energy to cut. Some cause less tissue damage than others (bipolar), but all cause at least a small zone of injury to tissue. Since there are no studies comparing the results (defined by successful pregnancy) of even the least damaging energy source to the results from using scissors, I personally prefer to avoid that risk by only using scissors to treat AS.

Office or Operating Room for Hysteroscopy?

There are a number of advantages to treatment in an office setting. It is far more convenient and less anxiety provoking than an operating room. The cost of an operating room in a hospital or outpatient surgical center is much greater than the cost of an office setting. This is a major factor if repeated procedures need to be done. Unless I expect severe adhesions or anticipate the need to insert a balloon I much prefer to do hysteroscopy in the office.

Basic diagnostic hysteroscopy can usually be done in an office setting with minimal discomfort using local anesthesia. I attach a video camera to the hystero-scope, so my patient can also see, and then insert the hysteroscope into the uterus under direct vision while using saline to fill the uterus. Women can typically carry out their normal activities for the rest of the day.

If I expect significant adhesions I will usually recommend intravenous analgesia and mild sedation for office hysteroscopy. If I plan to use abdominal ultrasound to help guide the procedure I will have the patient leave her bladder full to avoid the need to use a catheter. Adhesions that are mostly near the cervix in the lower portion of the uterus can usually be easily freed in this setting, avoiding the need for a general anesthetic and the expense of an operating room. To keep these adhesions from reforming I will have the patient come in and with the cervix numbed pass a small dilator into the uterus. This can also be done by her local gynecologist if she is from out of the area. Since the upper part of uterus is normal the prognosis is excellent (figure 2).

If little endometrium shows up on a vaginal probe ultrasound I would anticipate severe adhesions in the upper part of the uterus. This would require a more lengthy procedure and more manipulation of the instruments than could be comfortably done in the office. In this case I would recommend doing the surgery in an operating room with anesthesia, again using transabdominal ultrasound guidance (figures 4a-c).

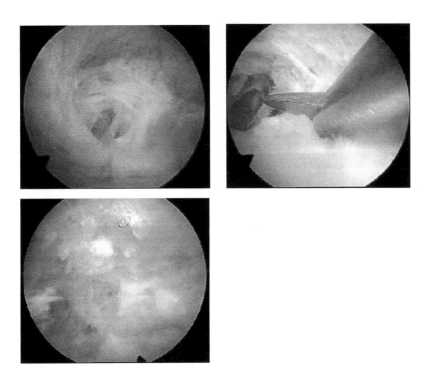

Figures 4a, 4b, 4c

Figure 4a: Adhesions involving entire uterus. Here lower uterine segment is completely blocked by adhesions.
Figure 4b: Adhesions in the lower segment are cut with hysteroscopic scissors. This is being done with ultrasound guidance in the operating room.
Figure 4c: The endometrial cavity is almost completely restored, but little endometrium is seen. A balloon should be placed. This patient was lost to follow-up so her outcome is not known.

Prevention of Recurrent Adhesions

What to do after the hysteroscopy is where another controversy begins. Two raw surfaces adjacent to each other usually stick together. At first there is just sticky "goo" holding things together. This is easily separated. With time fibrous tissue grows in which acts like strong glue. An example I like to use is to imagine a bad burn of a hand and fingers. If it is bandaged so the fingers are together, and left like that for weeks, the fingers will be stuck together when the bandage is removed. How do we prevent that from happening? For the hand we change dressings and move the fingers around frequently so they don't stick together. How do we do that to the inside of the uterus?

One option is to leave a mechanical barrier in the uterus until it is healed enough to cover the raw surfaces. A "foley" catheter is designed to drain the bladder and can be used if the tip is cut off, but the balloon is round and not matched to the shape of the uterus. I prefer to use the Cook "balloon" when treating adhesions near the top corners of the uterus because the shape conforms to the uterus and it needs little inflation to stay in place. It's helpful to use the ultrasound to guide and confirm correct placement. Patients are treated with antibiotics as well as estrogens, and it is left in for 7-10 days.

The second option is to mechanically separate the walls of the uterus, just as we would do the fingers of our hand example. The simplest way to do this is to place a small probe or dilator through the cervix into the uterus and sweep it back and forth. If the adhesions were just in the lower portion of the uterus repeating this for several weeks in a row usually prevents recurrence. If there are adhesions in the upper uterus we can do a hysteroscopy a week or two after the initial treatment or after removing the balloon if one has been placed. This allows assessment of the results, regrowth of endometrium, and cutting of any recurrent adhesions under direct vision. Typically this would be repeated on a regular basis until the uterus has healed. The largest barrier to repeated hysteroscopy is the cost, especially if the procedure requires a full operating room. The cost is greatly reduced by doing hysteroscopy in the office.

Although there are no studies on repeat hysteroscopy for AS, there is a small study on using repeat hysteroscopy to reduce adhesions after hysteroscopic removal of fibroids on opposing walls — a situation at high risk for adhesion formation. Nine such women had an IUD placed after treatment and 7 of the 9 were noted to have adhesions at follow-up hysteroscopy. The next 7 women with opposing myomas had office hysteroscopy 1 to 2 weeks after the resection. All 7 were noted to have adhesions, which were easily lysed with the tip of the hysteroscope. At follow-up hysteroscopy, all of the women remained free of adhesions. The numbers are small and the results after fibroid removal may be different than for AS. Nevertheless, the risks of office hysteroscopy are low and the study did show a significant benefit.

So which method of preventing adhesion reformation is best? Ideally we would have a barrier we could leave in the uterus at the time of surgery which doesn't need to be removed. Since we have to do *something*, we are forced to make decisions without any studies comparing the balloon to repeat hysteroscopy. So here is what makes sense to me, but understand that there are no good studies comparing techniques.

1. Since adhesions near the cervix can easily be prevented by passing a dilator through the cervix, I don't see the need to leave in a balloon.

2. Moderate adhesions, in which the upper corners of the uterus are relatively intact can easily be freed during office hysteroscopy. If the original hysteroscopy was done in the office, then I usually do a repeat

hysteroscopy in 1 to 2 weeks. Is this better than using a balloon? That hasn't been tested, but since I wouldn't try to insert a Cook balloon in the office, it's only an option if the initial hysteroscopy is done in the office.

3. I treat severe adhesions and those expected to be in the upper corners of the uterus in the operating room, where I can also place a Cook balloon. In this situation the balloon makes sense and I will use it. I also like to do an office hysteroscopy several weeks after removing the balloon. Again, there is not scientific proof that this is beneficial.

On an encouraging note, studies are being done on preventing adhesions after surgery by infusing a woman's stem into the uterus to encourage regrowth of endometrium. Other compounds to reduce adhesion reformation are also being studied, and hopefully will reduce the need for balloons and repeat hysteroscopy.

Preventing Asherman's Syndrome

It is important to recognize situations that are high risk for the development of AS. At times an emergency D&C may be required and even lifesaving in the case of severe hemorrhage. At particularly high risk is a situation with retained tissue after a miscarriage, delivery, or abortion. This can be treated medically at times, but if it persists can often be removed under direct vision through a hysteroscope rather than by D&C. This avoids trauma to normal tissues. The use of estrogens should also be considered. Liberal use of follow-up office hysteroscopy can break up early adhesions before they become fibrous.

Myomectomy, the removal of fibroids, can result in adhesions if fibroids are removed from the endometrial cavity. Figure 5a shows a central adhesion, seen at office hysteroscopy done ten weeks after an abdominal myomectomy during which multiple fibroids were removed from the walls of the uterus and in the cavity of the uterus. Figure 5b shows a normal uterine cavity after cutting the adhesion at the time of office hysteroscopy.

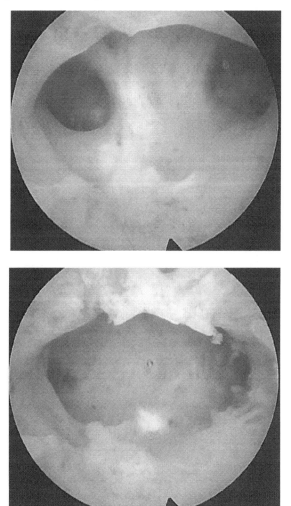

Figures 5a and 5b

Figure 5a: Office hysteroscopy done ten weeks after an abdominal myomectomy during which multiple fibroids were removed from the walls of the uterus and inside the uterus.

Figure 5b: Normal endometrial cavity after cutting the adhesion at the time of office hysteroscopy. The patient conceived three months later and had a normal pregnancy.

Hysteroscopic removal of fibroids is another procedure that can cause adhesions, especially if the fibroids are on opposite sides of the uterus. Determining which fibroids should be removed hysteroscopically and which should be treated by another approach requires extensive experience in treating fibroids. Likewise this type of specialized surgery should only be done by an experienced hysteroscopic surgeon doing it on a regular basis. I don't hesitate to do a follow-up office hysteroscopy to be sure no adhesions are forming.

In summary, hysteroscopy is the gold standard for the diagnosis and treatment of Asherman's syndrome. The best way to prevent recurrent adhesions after initial treatment is still controversial, and new methods are being developed. Many hysteroscopic procedures can safely be done in an office setting, thus avoiding the cost of an operating room.

32. KEITH ISAACSON, M.D.

Since 1989, I have seen, treated and gotten to know hundreds of patients diagnosed with scar tissue in the uterine or cervical canal. While each patient is unique, the common theme to each newly diagnosed condition is frustration. Most patients are frustrated about the mere existence of the condition (likely having heard about it for the first time), the common misdiagnosis of the condition for months or years by their health care providers, the lack of uniformity of treatment and the high rate of recurrence after treatment. As a clinician I want to state up front that I share these same frustrations. It has been well documented in the OB/GYN literature that there is a risk of developing intrauterine scar tissue following any trauma to the uterine cavity. These risks are small in uncomplicated D&C's done for first trimester miscarriages and are much higher in patients undergoing postpartum D&C for retained placenta or multiple fibroid resections within the uterine cavity. Physicians are aware of these risks and patients should be informed as well. This is not to say that the D&C is inappropriately performed. The point is to educate the patient of all known risks of a procedure so the condition may be recognized and treated promptly.

As early as 2005, I submitted a manuscript to a leading gynecology surgery journal about a novel technique to treat Asherman's Syndrome[4]. The technique involves diagnosing and treating intrauterine scar tissue in the office with no anesthesia and following up with these patients at 2 and 6 weeks post procedure instead of placing an intrauterine stint or balloon. The patients in my study had developed Asherman's Syndrome as a result of

---

[4] In this chapter, I will refer to any amount of intrauterine scar tissue as Asherman's Syndrome. True Asherman's Syndrome, however, refers to patients who not only have scar tissue but no menses as well.

postpartum D&Cs, first trimester D&Cs, prior fibroid removal surgeries and Cesarean sections. Initially, the manuscript was rejected. The reviewer commented that it is common knowledge that the only procedure a patient can develop intrauterine scar tissue from is a postpartum D&C. This lack of knowledge from a supposed "expert" in our field is sadly not isolated. When I see this degree of ignorance from the experts in our field, I'm not surprised that so many health care providers across the globe are unaware of how frequently intrauterine scar tissue occurs. Because most women breastfeed their newborns, it is not uncommon for no menses to occur until the baby is weaned. This is often 6-18 months after a postpartum D&C and the obstetrician or gynecologist neglects to consider Asherman's as a cause for no menses or amenorrhea. When a woman who has undergone a D&C has cyclic symptoms such as pain without vaginal bleeding, Asherman's Syndrome should be the first diagnosis to consider.

Despite the frequent misdiagnosis of Asherman's Syndrome, it is easily diagnosed with in office procedures such as saline infusion sonography or office hysteroscopy. During these tests, there is no excuse for missing the diagnosis in patients with a typical clinical history, i.e. prior uterine procedure along with a change in menstrual flow that is either light or non-existent. However, contrary to common feeling, the reason the scar tissue developed in the first place is rarely due to an inappropriate procedure. If a patient is hemorrhaging after a delivery, a D&C is the right procedure to save the uterus and the patient's life. In a first trimester miscarriage, D&C is an option but there are other options such as watchful waiting and medical therapies that should be discussed. These options have the downside of delaying therapy even though they are less invasive and have a smaller risk of scar tissue development. If a fibroid has to be removed due to bleeding and anemia, it is appropriate to use the best surgical technique to minimize the risk of scar tissue but we will never reduce that risk to zero. The best technique means that two opposing fibroids in the cavity should not be operated on in one procedure. The two cut edges will stick together. Often patients are upset and angry and feel that the initial procedure that led to the scar tissue was fouled in some way. My experience is that mishandling is rarely the cause of Asherman's. Until we know the real cause for Asherman's, we have a hard time preventing it. The question should be asked as to whether or not the same condition that caused a retained placenta is one that places the patient at risk for intrauterine scar tissue.

Once Asherman's Syndrome is diagnosed, should the adhesions be treated with scissors, electrical energy, morcellators, another D&C? Understandably, the lack of uniform techniques among surgeons is another source of frustration. Unfortunately, we do not yet have definitive randomized controlled trials to guide us to the best technique with the most favorable outcome. Surgeons have to use their best judgment and experience. I prefer using cold scissors and my colleague may prefer electrical energy. I choose this because I believe that cold scissors is the best technique that will not cause any thermal damage to nearby surrounding endometrium. As well, I can be aggressive with small scissors and not be concerned with a burn injury to bowel or bladder. No surgeon has proof that one technique is superior to the other. How can the patient decide if the surgeons don't even agree? The surgeon needs to clearly explain why he or she is suggesting a particular method of surgical therapy over another. If the explanation makes sense to the patient, then the patient should proceed. If the surgeon says "this is how I've always done it" or "this is how what I learned fifteen years ago," the patient should get another opinion.

The final source of frustration for the patient and the clinician is that intrauterine scar tissue will recur to some degree more often than not. How do we attempt to minimize the risk of recurrence? Described in the literature are mechanical methods to keep the uterine walls apart such as IUDs and balloons as well as hormonal regimens to promote healing such as high dose estrogen. A recently described technique is a follow-up up office hysteroscopic procedure to break up any scar tissue while it is reforming and before it becomes thick and permanent. As you might expect, there are no studies comparing one post procedure regimen to another and therefore we cannot conclude that one surgeon's post procedure recommendation is any better or worse than another's. Again, a thorough dialogue between the surgeon and the patient is key to reducing this source of patient frustration. The surgeon needs to help the patient understand why he or she is recommending hormones or balloons or repeat hysteroscopic procedures. My preference is to cut the adhesions in the office with small cold scissors. I then place the patient on oral estrogen for 30 days. I recommend a follow-up hysteroscopy at two weeks and 6 weeks. By 6 weeks, the cavity is healed and the results are known.

Because of all of the misinformation, frustration and confusions, I spend a good deal of time with the patients I see suffering with Asherman's Syndrome. Our conversations typically result in a bond, a partnership with a high level of mutual respect. Beginning with the initial visit, we discuss the reason the condition exists, the prior efforts for treating the condition, the options for future treatment, the goals for success and the likelihood of achieving those goals. Goals for patients may be to achieve a successful pregnancy, eliminate cyclic pain or have her cycles return to normal. Because there are many reasonable choices for treatment, I will actually encourage each patient to get a second or third opinion before she selects one that makes the most sense to her. I know the patient will be most comfortable with her outcome, whether good or bad, when she is well informed and an active participant in the decision making process.

Fortunately, Asherman's is not a life threatening disease. Unfortunately, such diseases never get the kind of research funding that diabetes, heart disease or breast cancer do. We have recently started a center for research, Center for Gynepathology Research (CGR) between my minimally invasive gynecology surgery practice at Harvard and the center for tissue engineering at the Massachusetts Institute of Technology (MIT). This center focuses on benign conditions in women that can lead to a great deal of suffering, i.e Asherman's Syndrome, endometriosis and uterine fibroids. Bringing brilliant minds from MIT to this field will no doubt lead to great advances. Our only limitation will be funding and we, like most researchers, are constantly looking for financial support for these efforts.

Getting to know patients, being able to work with them to manage their medical problems is what attracts me to the field of medicine. This exchange is often heightened with Asherman's patients because most are well informed and motivated. I very much enjoy working together on this problem. Having said that, I would trade all the respectful relationships and friendships I have made with patients with Asherman's for a single cure with more predictable and reliable results.

33. CHARLES MARCH, M.D.

DECONSTRUCTING THE MYTHS ABOUT ASHERMAN'S SYNDROME: A FORTY-TWO-YEAR-PERSPECTIVE

As early as 1950, Dr. Joseph G. Asherman wrote in the *Journal of Obstetrics and Gynecology of the British Empire* about the condition that now bears his name: "It is neither sufficiently understood nor appreciated that uterine curettage, especially repeated curettage, leaves traces which have far-reaching consequences for the patient." Uterine curettage (typically a D&C) and other common uterine surgeries may damage the lining of the uterus or endometrium and/or lead to intrauterine adhesions (IUA), bridges of scar tissue that cause the uterine walls to stick together. In normal pregnancies, about a week after fertilization occurs, an embryo implants into the uterine lining and therein finds nutrients for growth. A damaged endometrium can prevent implantation of the embryo or cause pregnancy loss or severe complications. The devastating consequences of Asherman's Syndrome (AS) thus include infertility, recurrent miscarriage, and complicated pregnancies. More than sixty years after Dr. Asherman's research, many doctors continue to reinforce myths about Asherman's Syndrome, leading to a frustrating delay in diagnosis and treatment. The patient loses money, irreplaceable time, and hope. The good news is that Asherman's *can* be anticipated, prevented, and treated in a methodical and comprehensive way. To do so, we must deconstruct the numerous myths about Asherman's Syndrome that exist.

Myth #1: Asherman's is rare.

In the 1970s, while in training, I was taught that during my career as a fertility specialist, I could expect to treat (at most) five patients with AS. To date, I am more than 2,000 patients above that estimate. Data in the chart below detail the prevalence of adhesions after uterine surgery and suggest that the incidence is increasing. Studies show that after a D&C performed because of pregnancy loss or retained products of conception, the incidence of Asherman's can be as high as 20 percent, 30 percent, or even 40 percent. In the case of repeated curettages, the incidence can be even higher. These data destroy all claims that AS is rare. Those who continue to subscribe to this archaic belief contribute to a delay in diagnosis and treatment. Furthermore, some doctors even state that some women are "scar formers." No data support this claim, and by invoking it, its proponents are simply blaming the patient. This claim is especially devastating for those who develop AS following a pregnancy termination.

Condition/Procedure	Percentage with adhesions	Reference
Amenorrhea	1.7	Am J Obstetrics & Gynecology (1964) 89:304
Infertility	1.5	Obstetrics & Gynecology (1969) 34:288–299
Infertility	4.0	Gynecol Obstet (1957) 56:521
Post-Cesarean section	2.8	J Gynecol/Obstet Biol Rep (1979) 8:723–726

Postpartum D&C (any time)	3.7	Acta Obstet/Gyn Scand Supp 4 (1961) 40:4
Postpartum D&C (2nd–4th week after delivery)	23.4	Danish Medical Bulletin (1960) 7:50-51
D&C performed soon after fetal demise detected	6.4	International J Fertility (1982) 27:117-118
D&C performed long after fetal demise detected	30.9	International J Fertility (1982) 27:117-118
Voluntary pregnancy termination	13	Ljubljana Abortion Study (1971–1973)
Recurrent spontaneous abortion	39	Rev Franc Gyn Obstet (1966) 61:550–552
Recurrent spontaneous abortion	48	Eur J Obstet Gynecol Reprod Biol (1994) 57:171
Retained products of conception	40	Human Reproduction (1998) 13:3347–3350
1 spontaneous abortion	16.3	Human Reproduction (1993) 8:442–444
2 spontaneous abortions	14	
3 spontaneous abortions	32	

Myth #2: Infection causes Asherman's.

Clinical infections are rare, having been present in less than one percent of my patients. Except for pelvic tuberculosis, which is almost exclusively a disease of those from developing nations, no other infectious agent causes endometrial destruction in the absence of uterine surgery.

Myth #3: Only an overaggressive D&C causes Asherman's.

Overaggressive curettage can cause AS, and unfortunately some gynecologists still curette until they hear and feel the "uterine cry" (an abrasive sound and gritty sensation detected when a sharp curette is scraped over uterine muscle stripped of its overlying endometrium). Currently, most curettages are performed blindly, that is, the doctor places a curette inside the uterus in order to remove the tissue, but he/she cannot see inside the uterus in order to accurately control its placement, action or judge when to cease curetting. Over the last few decades, some physicians have begun to perform this type of surgery using hysteroscopic or ultrasound guidance, which allows the doctor greater control over the procedure. Nevertheless, *any* curettage can cause Asherman's. Believing otherwise only stymies early diagnosis and treatment. If a physician believes this myth, and also sees himself/herself as a careful physician, he/she will often conclude that the patient could not have developed AS from the curettage, and that her problem must be related to a hormonal problem or to stress. Furthermore, many believe that Asherman's arises only from the use of a "sharp" curette, not a suction curette. No data exist to support this belief, and review of operative reports from AS patients negates the claim.

Though many believe that Asherman's comes only from pregnancy-related surgeries, myomectomy (removal of one or more fibroid tumors), metroplasty (for the treatment of a congenital uterine division), and "diagnostic" D&C can all give rise to AS. In fact, the frequency of IUA occurring after uterine surgery *unassociated* with a pregnancy is rising more rapidly than that of all other causes. Unfortunately, IUAs following these procedures is the most difficult to treat.

Myth #4: Patients with Asherman's don't get their monthly periods.

Although 93 % of my patients with AS have had scanty or no periods before treatment, the remainder have had painless menses of normal flow and duration, including 2.5 % of those who were diagnosed with severe intrauterine scarring. Many physicians quibble over terminology, proclaiming, "She gets her period, so she doesn't have AS," or, "only part of her uterine cavity is scarred; she doesn't have AS unless the entire cavity is scarred." While the purist may desire a crystal clear definition of AS with strict criteria, we do not have one, we will not, and we cannot. Many of us prefer the term "intrauterine adhesions"; although more clear and more descriptive, this term also has limitations. Patients with surface deficiencies of the endometrium (without fibrous bridges to the opposing uterine wall) are adhesion free, but suffer the same conditions as do those patients with adhesions. Thus, although affixing the eponym "Asherman's" to this diverse condition invites justifiable complaints, the term "Asherman's Syndrome" signifies a range of acquired endometrial deficiencies and their significant consequences of menstrual aberrations, infertility, recurrent pregnancy loss, and complicated pregnancies. If a woman detects a reduction in, or loss of, menstruation after uterine surgery, and other possible causes such as hormonal imbalance are eliminated via blood tests, she should insist on one of three simple diagnostic tests to see if she has Asherman's Syndrome. They are: 1) diagnostic hysteroscopy, during which a small telescope affixed to a camera is inserted into the uterus; 2) hysterosalpingogram (HSG), an X-ray test in which an iodine dye is inserted into the uterus in order to outline it and the fallopian tubes; or 3, a saline infusion sonogram (SIS, hydrosonogram or hysterosonogram), an ultrasound study of the uterus performed while sterile saline in instilled via the cervix. Of the three, diagnostic hysteroscopy is the most conclusive way to determine the presence of Asherman's and to determine its severity, because the telescope provides a direct view of the inside of the uterus.

Myth #5: The consequences of Asherman's Syndrome are limited to reproductive problems. If you don't plan to get pregnant, there's no reason to treat it.

Those women with amenorrhea and some of those who have scanty menstrual flow often have scarring that is limited to the upper cervix or lower portion of the uterus. If there is functioning endometrium above the site of obstruction, the patient may experience intense pain every month because her menstrual flow cannot exit via the cervix and therefore is partially "trapped," trying to exit via the narrow openings leading to her fallopian tubes. If treatment is not undertaken in a timely fashion, this refluxed menstrual flow may lead to the development of endometriosis, a painful condition where endometrial-like cells grow in other parts of the body.

Myth #6: Asherman's is not treatable.

We use a multipronged approach for the treatment of Asherman's Syndrome:

GOALS	METHODS
• Repair uterine cavity	• Adhesiolysis using microscissors under direct hysteroscopic visualization.
• Prevent re-scarring	• Intrauterine stent placement for between 1 and 4 weeks with the concomitant administration of an antibiotic.
• Promote healing	• High-dose estrogen therapy
• Diagnostic follow-up (uterine architecture)	• Diagnostic hysteroscopy, hysterosalpingogram (HSG) or saline infusion sonogram (SIS)
• Diagnostic follow-up (uterine function)	• Mid-cycle ultrasound of the endometrium

Depending upon the initial cause, normal uterine architecture may be restored in up to ninety percent of patients, usually after a single surgical procedure. A comprehensive approach to treatment involves:

1) meticulous hysteroscopic surgery using micro scissors;

2) stent placement to reduce the frequency of scar re-formation;

3) high-dose estrogen therapy to encourage endometrial growth and healing;

4) confirmation of cure before permitting the patient to try to conceive; and

5) ongoing surveillance of all pregnancies up to and including delivery. This approach has been demonstrated to optimize outcome. Among those who have suffered repeated spontaneous pregnancy loss, a comprehensive evaluation of the couple to detect other possible causes for repeated miscarriage is mandatory.

The superiority of hysteroscopic treatment was proven in the early 1970s. Sadly, even in 2016, some doctors use traumatic blind curettage, the same procedure that caused the IUA, to treat it! Others follow hysteroscopic treatment with curettage to "remove" the cut scars. These approaches are unnecessary and usually cause more damage. Furthermore, during the decades we have compiled extensive data that demonstrate convincingly that treatment of IUA with a laser or with electrosurgical instruments is less effective than treatment with micro scissors. Because adhesions do *not* bleed when cut, the use of any energy source to "cauterize" the cut is unnecessary. Additionally, among those who require multiple surgeries, the use of energy inside the uterus during any single surgery is associated with a poorer prognosis.

My initial experience with operative hysteroscopy was in 1970, and I have performed more than ten thousand procedures since then. In 2001, the

American Association of Gynecologic Laparoscopists awarded me the title of "Pioneer in Hysteroscopy" for my development of new treatment regimens for patients with uterine abnormalities and Asherman's Syndrome; six years earlier I had developed a balloon stent that could be inserted into the uterus to prevent further scarring following reproductive surgery. Serum may ooze from the areas of the freshly dissected scars and promote scars to re-form; the nonreactive stent in the uterus keeps the uterine walls from touching one another during the postoperative period. We use the Cook Balloon Uterine Stent, a silicone sac which is filled with saline after it is placed in the uterus. Because of its triangular shape, this device conforms to the shape of the normal uterus. Depending on the severity of the case, the woman may have the stent placed in her uterus for up to four weeks, and I prescribe antibiotics for the duration of the stent placement. There are other devices on the market that are used as stents. It should be noted that no randomized controlled studies are available that compare one device to another, or to stent placement compared to the use of no stent.

Other doctors prefer to perform multiple hysteroscopies early in the postoperative period to verify normal healing and, if needed, to cut re-forming scars before they become dense. Again, clinical trials are needed to determine if one method of postoperative management is superior to the others. The use of high-dose estrogen therapy to promote endometrial overgrowth and healing is standard practice.

Although it appears to be "common sense," the practice of performing follow-up tests to ensure that the uterus is ready for pregnancy after treatment is still not routine. When asked about follow-up tests, the authors of two studies (Obstet Gynecol 1976; 47:701–705; Obstet Gynecol 1986; 67: 864–867), which warned of the dire outcomes of pregnancies which followed therapy for IUA, indicated that usually the cavity was not rechecked prior to recommending that conception be attempted. Furthermore, even if the uterus was persistently abnormal, patients were advised to attempt pregnancy rather than be offered another surgery. It seems like a no-brainer to me: following removal of adhesions via hysteroscopic surgery, I have always checked the cavity by HSG or in-office hysteroscopy. If an HSG is the follow-up method, the reproductive surgeon who performed the surgery should personally review the X-ray films him/herself. Hysteroscopy offers the advantage of permitting further cutting of scars if there has been a partial recurrence. If these follow-up tests come back normal, the doctor should perform a mid-cycle ultrasound to determine endometrial growth and quality.

Myth #7: Pregnancies that occur after treatment are doomed.

Most pregnancies are successful, *if* the uterus has been repaired successfully. To optimize success, these pregnancies should be monitored closely. This monitoring takes two paths: one is related specifically to the AS and the other is not. Many women with AS have had recurrent pregnancy loss. Although the diagnosis of IUA may have been made only after multiple spontaneous miscarriages, the scarring may have developed after the initial miscarriage and curettage, after the last D&C, or at some point in between. Although the association between AS and recurrent miscarriage is clear, the inability to determine the onset of the AS with certainty mandates that all those with AS who have suffered multiple pregnancy losses undergo a complete investigation, rather than assuming that the intrauterine scarring has been the cause. A combination of delayed childbearing, multiple losses, and a delay in establishing the diagnosis of AS often results in post-AS pregnancies occurring in women who are somewhat older and may have hormonal deficiencies that will require supplementation during early pregnancy. Therefore, such monitoring is vitally important.

Myth #8: If a post-AS pregnancy progresses beyond the first trimester, all is fine.

Many of those with AS have had multiple uterine procedures and surgeries and therefore multiple forced cervical dilations; consequently, they are at increased risk for an "incompetent" or weakened cervix. The physical pressure of the growing fetus, placenta, and amniotic fluid on a weakened cervix may cause the cervix to open before the baby is ready to be born, leading to second-trimester loss or preterm labor. Frequent ultrasound monitoring of the cervix to measure cervical length and of the fetal membranes to detect "funneling" can detect early changes, signaling the need for cervical cerclage (stitching the cervix closed during pregnancy).

Placenta accreta, an abnormal, densely adherent attachment of the placenta to the uterine wall (on occasion, even into and through the wall), also occurs more often with AS patients, particularly in those who had prior damage to the basal endometrium. For those who have had placenta accreta previously and for those who are at high risk for this complication should undergo an MRI in the late second trimester in order to detect this condition. Despite its accuracy, an MRI is not perfect and therefore, for those who are at high risk for placenta accreta, we recommend that delivery be planned to occur on a weekday morning, when the hospital, laboratory, blood bank, operating room and interventional radiology are fully staffed, should complications arise. Even if delivery of the infant and placenta progresses smoothly and even if visual inspection of the placenta suggest that it is complete, manual exploration of the uterus allows assurance that there are no retained fragments and allows prompt removal if the opposite is true.

Although intrauterine growth restriction (IUGR), a situation where the fetus is unusually small, has occurred only three times among the more than 1,000 successful pregnancies which have occurred in my patients, this condition has been reported to be more frequent among those who conceive after treatment of AS. It is believed that endometrial deficiency can hinder placental development, leading to growth restriction of the fetus. In more severe cases, IUGR increases the risk of motor and neurological disabilities in the fetus or fetal death.

Myth #9: Asherman's cannot be anticipated or prevented.

Obviously, the first key is to anticipate who may develop AS. At highest risk are those who have been treated for recurrent loss by repeated curettage, and those who undergo curettage any time during the second to the fourth week after the delivery.

If faced with miscarriage (intrauterine fetal demise), surgical evacuation may not be necessary. If the loss occurs early in the pregnancy, the physician should consider the use of the drug misoprostol (Cytotec), which causes uterine contractions to aid evacuation. The drug should be taken shortly after fetal demise is detected, because its success rate decreases as the interval between fetal demise and its use increases. If curettage is required, it too should be performed as soon as possible, because the likelihood of adhesions following surgery increases as the time between fetal demise and D&C is prolonged. If curettage is necessary, it must be done under ultrasound guidance.

Women who have retained products of conception (RPOC) after a prior delivery, those with a prior complicated delivery, and those who have undergone therapy for AS are at the highest risk for partial placental retention and the uterus *must* be explored manually immediately after vaginal delivery. Even the most meticulous inspection of the placenta may fail to detect its "incompleteness," and a fragment or an accessory lobe of the placenta may remain in the uterus, which can cause hemorrhage and lead to subsequent curettage. If hemorrhage occurs during delivery, the obstetrician has a "golden" opportunity to make the diagnosis of RPOC by immediately exploring the uterus manually. This uterine exploration permits removal of any placental fragments; if bleeding occurs days or weeks later, curettage is not necessary because the physician knows that RPOC cannot be the cause. Alternately, if only *delayed* postpartum hemorrhage occurs, ultrasound can detect retained products of conception. If the ultrasound data suggests retained products of conception, again the use of pharmaceuticals *may* cause their evacuation, averting the need for curettage.

When D&C is absolutely necessary in any of these cases, prophylactic measures against the development of adhesions, *similar to the ones we use to treat Asherman's,* are surely worth taking, including curettage under ultrasound guidance or RPOC removal under hysteroscopic control, intravenous antibiotics, intrauterine stent placement, and high-dose estrogen therapy. Furthermore, postpartum patients who are breast-feeding remain estrogen deficient for a prolonged time, and thus the stimulus to endometrial regeneration is absent. The estrogen-deficient environment during or after pregnancy has been reported to increase the risk of uterine adhesion formation. Recommending that nursing be discontinued while prescribing estrogen treatment may be of value. Although I have made these recommendations for many years and believe them to pose no harm and to be effective, we need more research and clinical trials to definitively prove their value.

With respect to uterine surgery in the non-pregnant patient, such as surgery for fibroid removal (whether hysteroscopic, laparoscopic, or by open abdomen), many surgeons prescribe a gonadotropin-releasing hormone agonist, such as leuprolide acetate (Lupron) or nafarelin acetate (Synarel), to reduce blood loss during surgery, reduce tumor size preoperatively, and/or to cause thinning of the endometrium, thereby affording a clearer view of the uterine interior. However, as the drug-induced atrophy of the endometrial surface progresses, the basal layer becomes more susceptible to damage during surgery. As an alternative, techniques such as delaying surgery until after the effects of such drug treatment have worn off, thereby allowing endometrial regrowth to begin, or not prescribing these types of medications and simply scheduling the surgery shortly after menses end, provide less traumatic fibroid removal and the same clear view.

Some women are born with a uterine septum, i.e., a division that partially or completely separates the uterus into two parts. This division may cause repeated miscarriage or very premature delivery and increases the chance of developing endometriosis. Incision of a uterine septum is best accomplished with scissors, not electrical or laser energy. Energy spreads beyond the point of application, and its use may cause IUA, a complication that we have seen on many occasions among patients treated in this manner. In contrast, IUAs have occurred only once in our own series of more than eight hundred uterine septum incisions using scissors. Hysteroscopic myomectomy is commonly performed with a resectoscope, which has an electrically- activated wire loop. The electrical energy spreads beyond the point of application and may cause extensive damage. By reducing the power settings and by making other adjustments to the equipment, this risk is reduced greatly. More recently, a morcellator which can be used to remove polyps, myomas or retained products of conception has been introduced. This instrument uses only mechanical rather than energy forces to accomplish tissue removal, thereby obviating the risk of collateral damage.

Conclusion

Women and doctors are no doubt indebted to new technologies in the treatment of fertility, but technology alone will not save a women's fertility. Common sense, meticulous action, and compassion should still be the physician's guiding principles. While expert surgeons perform the initial studies on new and improved surgical instruments to prove safety and effectiveness, after these instruments are marketed, they are often used by doctors with little training, resulting in more damaged uteri. Furthermore, with the advent of in vitro fertilization (IVF) and the increasing number of women able to serve as gestational surrogates, the emphasis upon meticulous reproductive surgery has diminished and consequently more uteri are damaged. Although the subspecialty of reproductive endocrinology and infertility has been well established for decades, many of these specialists perform little or no reconstructive pelvic surgery, leaving these procedures to general gynecologists who have even less training and/or experience. All too often, many surgeons and general gynecologists subscribe to the thinking that "there is always IVF or surrogacy," putting the days of meticulous reproductive surgery behind them. Though these advances are miraculous in many cases, they are certainly not for all women: they can be financially prohibitive and emotionally and physically draining. Women should turn to these technologies as a last resort, not a first. Through further research and clinical studies, I hope the medical community will focus on awareness and best surgical practices and reverse the disturbing trend of the increasing incidence of Asherman's Syndrome.

34. DAVID L. OLIVE, M.D.

THINGS I HAVE COME TO BELIEVE

My foray into the world of Asherman's Syndrome began roughly 15 years ago and was a complete accident. I was in a teaching institution. We had an interesting patient and no one was sure exactly what to do to treat optimally. Being the evidence-based academician that I was, I scoured the medical literature in an attempt to discern the best approach. What I found was a whole gamut of uncontrolled trials, clinical opinion, and contradictory dogmas. It was an eye-opening experience.

Over the years I have treated over 300 women with all degrees of this disease, yet I have resisted publishing due to my fear of simply perpetuating the aforementioned problems. I could never hope to design and implement a high quality study with the low volume I was seeing, and the clinical issues were so numerous it felt like the "experts" in the field could never come to a consensus as to what the one or two key questions were. So I simply practiced, did my best, and critiqued what little literature there was on the subject.

However, I believe the time has now come to put my opinions into print...for the simple reason that I see so many women with Asherman's given what I believe to be very bad advice. To this end, I have listed 10 points I would like to make to the community of physicians and patients interested in this disease.

1. **Treatment of Asherman's Syndrome is not difficult.**

   Over the years I believe I have become an excellent endoscopist, and I frequently deal with extraordinarily difficult situations for minimally invasive surgery. However, hysteroscopic treatment of Asherman's

Syndrome is not one of them. With reasonably good hysteroscopic equipment and a fair ultrasonographer, truly efficacious surgery can be performed. The difficult aspects of the procedure reside in the surgeon's head, not his/her hands.

2. Electrosurgical instruments can be used.

The original dogma I was taught, in the hospital where I served as a resident, was that electrosurgery should never be used for intrauterine synechiae otherwise known as adhesions aka Asherman's. The thought was that tissue destruction was too great, and the resulting ischemia (inadequate blood supply) only led to adhesion reformation at a very high rate. However, this was when the only hysteroscopic electrosurgery was low wattage monopolar current. The recent advent of high wattage monopolar vaporization and bipolar electrosurgery has altered this premise. In the light of these technological advances it appears that electrosurgery can be safe and effective in the setting of treating such synechiae. At the Institute where I know practice, we utilize all types of instruments and energy sources to treat this disease, depending upon the situation. Thus, in any given case we may use blunt dissection initially, followed by incision with scissors, and finally bipolar incision to further open a densely scarred cavity and create an appropriate contour.

Limited medical publications, as well as my own experience and results, suggest this is a reasonable and effective approach.

3. **Laparoscopy is not necessary; ultrasound guidance is preferable.**

In cases of severe Asherman's Syndrome, my training had been to perform simultaneous laparoscopy for guidance. However, the only guidance this provided was confirmation that the uterus had been perforated by my hysteroscopic instruments. An epiphany occurred for me when I saw a video by Dr. Stephen Corson on the treatment of the disease with ultrasound-guided hysteroscopy. I immediately began using this technique, and have not looked back since. With our operative hysteroscopies for Asherman's, we routinely insert 500 ml of saline into the bladder via catheter, and then clamp the catheter to hold in the fluid. This enables abdominal ultrasonography to provide a very clear picture of the surgical proceedings. Ultrasonographic guidance makes much more sense, enabling me to see where I am in the uterus, how thick the wall is where I am working, and if any anomalous situations exist. My surgical goal, to create a cavity that is one centimeter from the serosal membrane surface fundally (top to bottom of the uterus) and laterally (side to side), is easily accomplished with ultrasound, but virtually impossible to attain with laparoscopic direction. In summary, laparoscopy is not helpful and expensive, as well as unnecessarily risky. I avoid it in any case that does not require the procedure for another indication.

4. **The primary goal is to keep the cavity open; endometrium repopulation (cell regrowth in the mucous membrane of uterus) is secondary.**

A certain researcher in his work at Yale, has shown quite nicely that bone marrow stem cells over time will migrate to the endometrium and repopulate the endometrial surface; this may be a few months or years, but it can occur. However, there must be a cavity to repopulate.

For this reason, my primary aim is always to create a cavity that will remain open for an extended time, regardless of the presence or absence of existing endometrium at the time of surgery. While it is nice if endometrium is present, and I try to never damage or destroy existing endometrium, its presence or absence is not a deal-breaker for whether or not I perform surgery or even the level of optimism of my post-surgical prognosis. Many patients have had no apparent endometrium, only to develop a near-normal cavity with a subsequent pregnancy 6-18 months later.

5. **Balloons are preferable to IUDs.**

The medical literature does contain a randomized trial stating this conclusion, but it also seems to make logical sense in this modern era: balloons can be made non-reactive and can be contoured to a variety of specifications, while intrauterine contraceptive devices are fixed in shape and material. Furthermore, an IUD is designed to be a local irritant, and works to prevent pregnancy by promoting local inflammation. This seems counter to the goals of surgery for intrauterine synechiae.

6. **A variety of balloons can and should be utilized for appropriate situations.**

The Cook Intrauterine Balloon stent is a valuable device that is shaped like a uterine cavity and can prevent re-adherence of raw surfaces within the uterus. It is a challenge to insert for many physicians, however, at my particular Institute, we have mastered insertion purely by trial and error: we now use a curved packing forcep to grasp a balloon wound tightly into a spiral while deflated. We then insert the instrument and balloon, while watching on abdominal ultrasound. Once positioned appropriately, a ring forcep is used to hold the stem in place while the packing forcep is carefully and gently removed. The balloon is then inflated, and the correct position confirmed by ultrasound.

A drawback of this balloon stent, however, is the relatively thin stem. The balloon is not an issue for cases of fundal adhesions at the top of the uterus or complete cavitary obliteration - where the uterus is completely unable to function due to adhesions. However, this device is woefully inadequate for Asherman's cases where the fundal cavity is intact but adhesions in the lower uterus cause outflow menstrual obstruction. In this situation, a 7-9 mm diameter foley catheter provides less likelihood of re-constriction in the outflow tract, maintaining a wide pathway from the cavity to the vagina. While care must be taken to not produce erosion of the fundal wall by the catheter tip beyond the balloon (I cut it off to avoid this complication occurring), the instrument is well suited for this particular version of Asherman's.

7. **Antibiotics are critically important while the balloon is in place.**

In all the years of performing surgery for Asherman's Syndrome, I have had only one bona fide disaster: a patient in whom a balloon stent was placed who neglected to take her antibiotics (and never told me when she developed a fever and pain). When a foreign object connects the sterile environment of the upper genital tract (uterine cavity) with the highly contaminated vagina, protection via antibiotic prophylaxis is imperative. When I leave stents in for 3-4 weeks, I instruct the patient to continue the prophylaxis antibiotic treatment throughout the timeframe to prevent the spread of infection to the uterus. I have yet to have a problem with infection when such a rule is adhered to.

8. **The postoperative hormonal protocol is as important as the surgery.**
Once a good cavity is created, it is imperative to give it the best chance possible to remain open. At the Fertility Institute where I practice, we frequently operate on patients with obliterated cavities. In this situation, we place a balloon stent for 4 weeks, and administer antibiotics and 8mg. oral estradiol daily. At the conclusion of the four weeks, we remove the stent, discontinue the antibiotics, and continue the estradiol. We also add medroxyprogesterone at this time. The estrogen and progestin are continued together for 2 weeks, and then stopped. Menses (menstrual bleeding) should begin in 2-3 days. Just after the conclusion of menses, an office hysteroscopy is performed to lyse (loosen) any reforming adhesions and to inspect the status of the cavity. Decisions regarding additional therapy are made at this time. This protocol is purely based upon trial and error; and I have to say it is the one that has given me the best results over the years.

9. **Office-based hysteroscopy is ideal.**
While the above protocol is what I use, it is not what I would consider optimal. The ideal protocol would follow my initial hysteroscopic opening of the cavity with office hysteroscopies every 4-7 days to lyse adhesions while in their early, formative stage. However, this approach becomes quite costly for the patient and equally our practice, as we often perform such procedures at or below cost. Furthermore, many patients are not local, and thus cannot hop over to

our office every few days. It is a rare patient for whom this ongoing observation and lysis of adhesions is a practical follow-up. Nevertheless, having at least one such office-based hysteroscopy provides essential information as to the effectiveness of the procedure, critical knowledge for the physician trying to develop skill and expertise and for the patient who needs to make decisions about future therapeutic options.

10. Deterioration of outcome can and often does occur with time.

I once believed that if, at the end of 6 weeks post-hysteroscopy the cavity remained open and adhesion-free, it would remain that way in perpetuity. This is definitely not the case. It has become apparent to me that some women will re-adhere months after their initial treatment and follow-up. For this reason, continued long term surveillance is critical for optimal patient outcomes as well as accurate self-assessment of suitability and viability of pregnancy occurring.

Despite the haphazard nature by which I entered this arena, I have truly enjoyed taking care of women with Asherman's Syndrome. Most afflicted women are a true challenge, and when the rewards occur they are substantial. In a gynecologic world where advice is quick to come from far too many practitioners that a hysterectomy is necessary, or the only alternative, I would contend that the pleasure of recreating that which has been lost far exceeds that of simple extirpation or removal. This, through my extensive practice and experience is what I have come to believe.

35. THIERRY VANCAILLIE, M.D. FRANZCOG

With twenty-five years of hindsight, I have many observations that affect how I treat this condition. Intra-uterine and, especially intra-cervical adhesions, are far more common than we first suspected and do occur without the traditional triad of pregnancy: the anti-estrogen status of a woman during pregnancy, a surgical procedure and the unsterile environment of the vagina and cervix which invite bacteria into the womb. As a matter of fact, almost every woman in menopause — which is a naturally occurring 'low estrogen environment' similar to pregnancy — will have intra-cervical adhesions in her uterus. These are frequently missed by those colleagues who routinely use cervical dilation prior to hysteroscopy. Even more interesting is the observation that women using long-term Progesterone for suppression of menses will develop intra-cervical and intra-uterine adhesions without any other known etiological factor in their history. The adhesions resulting from progesterone treatment are easily ruptured by blunt dissection and rarely become dense, nonetheless these observations are important and need to be factored in our approach to management.

My overall interpretation of these observations is that: 1] The development of intra-cervical and intra-uterine scarring is a natural 'aging' phenomenon of the uterus, possibly related to a chronic low-level inflammation associated with the vagina (it should be noted that estrogen appears to protect against the development of adhesions), 2] progesterone is deleterious, possibly because of its inherent anti-estrogen effect and 3] good vascularization is important in preventing adhesions from developing.

Prevention

As a result of these observations, treatment for my patients has included strict adherence to a protocol that aims to achieve the following:

1. Intervene during the proliferative phase of the cycle (= avoiding Progesterone) and support the healing after treatment with a high dose of estrogen for three weeks after intervention without Progesterone.

2. Provide antibiotic cover during the surgery and the immediate healing phase. For more than fifteen years, I have used Doxycycline because of the fact that this antibiotic accumulates in epithelial tissues (hence its use for treatment of Acne) and can therefore be started several days prior to the surgery. This means that the antibiotic will be there where it needs to be at the time of surgery.

3. Avoid vaso-constrictive agents, such as local anesthetics with Adrenaline during surgery, as they may cause tissue damage by anoxia. Ideally, I would like to add a local vaso-dilator during the healing phase after surgery, but have not been able to find a satisfactory product yet.

Treatment

Treatment of Asherman's Syndrome consists first of identifying pockets of normal uterine cavity and normal cervical canal and then, removal of the scar tissue in between these pockets. Imaging is important before and during surgery. The recent advances in sonography make it relatively simple to identify the presence of endometrium within the uterus. A careful sonographic inspection will guide the surgeon during the upcoming procedure. During the actual procedure I favor the use of X-Ray, although in recent times, both modalities have been used. The advantage of sonography is that the myometrium can be easily distinguished from the endometrium, whereas, X-Ray will provide information on the status of tubal patency. The use of a Tuohy type needle to identify pockets of normal cavity has been well described in other publications and is not the subject of this treatise.

Blunt dissection with scissors or the bevel of the hysteroscope will handle the majority of the adhesions. Unless dense avascular scar is present, there is no need to actually 'resect' or remove tissue. Occasionally, especially at the level of the isthmus and internal cervical os, the scarring can be quite dense. Removing the hard core of the scar tissue at that level should be a consideration and can be achieved with simple mechanical scissors. Only in rare circumstances is it necessary to use more aggressive equipment, such as a resectoscope with an electro-surgical cutting loop or knife.

In our experience at my medical practice, a surgical procedure for the treatment of Asherman's Syndrome should not exceed one hour. Perhaps better stated, if no progress is achieved within that period of time, it is unlikely that any will be achieved at all. Experience tells us that it is preferable to stop and re-schedule. In the intervening time interval between procedures, high dose estrogen may be considered to possibly facilitate the next intervention. We do warn patients that treatment of the condition may require multiple interventions.

At the end of the intervention, we now use a Hyaluronic Acid based gel to reduce the likelihood of recurrence of the adhesions. This gel remains in place for approximately five days and is slowly absorbed by the body. An obvious advantage of using a gel as an adhesion barrier is that it does not need to be removed. There is an initial clinical impression that using gel reduces the number of interventions needed to achieve a good outcome.

Recovery and Conception

Patients are told that once they have experienced a normal menstrual episode, they can proceed with attempts to conceive. When we suspect residual adhesions are present, we discourage patients from proceeding with conception, because we do not know how these adhesions may affect the subsequent pregnancy.

Pregnancy post-treatment of patients with Asherman's Syndrome should be considered high-risk. The issue is that the placenta in a woman with AS interacts differently with the uterine wall than a normal uterine wall. All pathology associated with the placenta (placental accreta and increta, but also growth retardation and preeclampsia) need to be anticipated as a potential complication of the subsequent pregnancy. A physician trained in high-risk obstetrics should follow anyone conceiving after treatment of Asherman's Syndrome.

A pregnancy post-Asherman treatment can, of course, fail. Should a miscarriage occur, we encourage a 'wait and see' attitude, allowing for the natural expulsion of products of conception. In those cases where an evacuation of products is needed, we will use a hysteroscopic approach to remove the residual placental tissue. In addition, we do initiate Estrogen treatment as soon as possible after evacuation. This is not based on scientific evidence, but rather on the concept that Estrogen does protect the uterine cavity and cervical canal from the formation of adhesions. We also encourage the use of antibiotics. Lactation possibly promotes the recurrence of intra-uterine scarring, but we do not go as far as recommending not to breastfeed because of the benefits to the baby.

Summary

There is a natural tendency for intra-uterine adhesions to recur. This observation underscores our belief that scar formation is a 'natural ageing phenomenon'. Based on my extensive clinical and research experience with this subject, I believe that a scarred uterus will age faster compared to a non-scarred uterus. To slow down this aging process, we encourage women who have been treated for Asherman's Syndrome and who want to keep the option of conceiving in the future, not to use any anti-estrogen type medication, such as the ever-present oral contraceptive pill. Obviously the observation of this tendency to recur also incites us to encourage women not to delay their attempt to conceive after successful treatment of their condition.

Made in the USA
Columbia, SC
20 November 2020